Growing
Self-Compassionate
Children

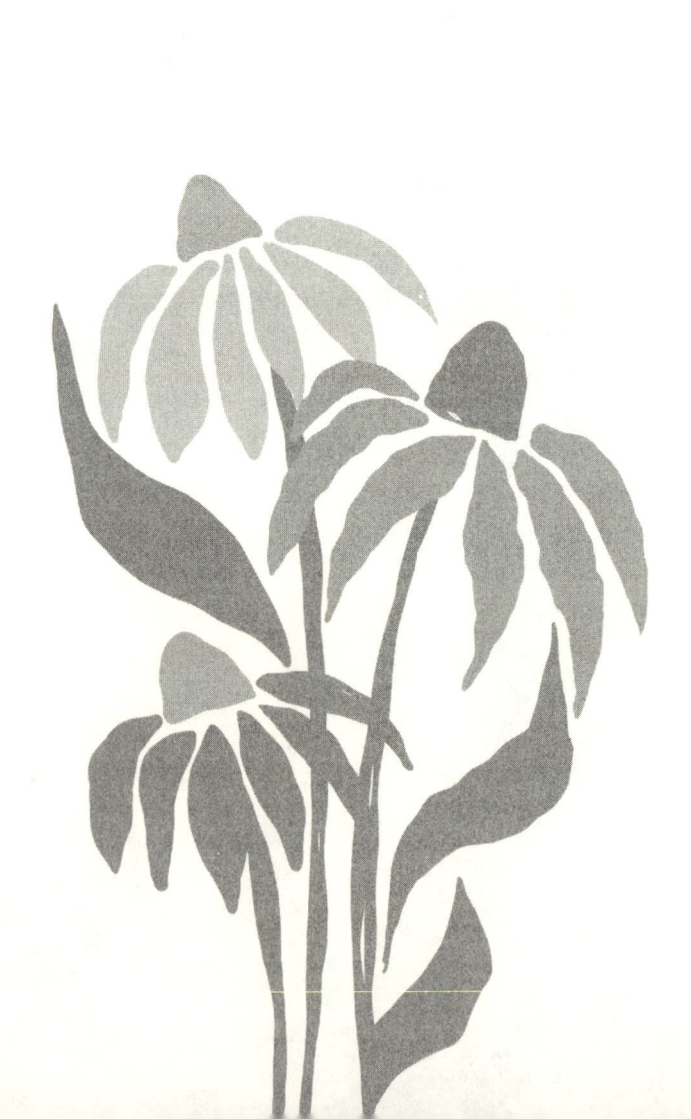

Growing
Self-Compassionate
Children

A Family Guide for
Nurturing Resiliency
and Kindness

WENDY O'LEARY
LOUISE SHANAGHER

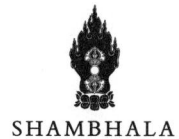

SHAMBHALA

Shambhala Publications, Inc.
2129 13th Street
Boulder, Colorado 80302
www.shambhala.com

Cover art: Mariya/Adobe Stock
Cover design: Daniel Urban-Brown
Interior design: Kate Huber-Parker

9 8 7 6 5 4 3 2 1

First Edition
Printed in the United States of America

Shambhala Publications makes every effort
to print on acid-free, recycled paper.
Shambhala Publications is distributed worldwide by
Penguin Random House, Inc., and its subsidiaries.

Library of Congress Cataloging-in-Publication Data

Names: O'Leary, Wendy, author. | Shanagher, Louise, author.
Title: Growing self-compassionate children: a family guide for nurturing
    resiliency and kindness / Wendy O'Leary, Louise Shanagher.
Description: First edition. | Boulder, Colorado: Shambhala, [2025] |
    Includes bibliographical references.
Identifiers: LCCN 2024016832 | ISBN 9781645473008 (trade paperback)
Subjects: LCSH: Self-acceptance in children. | Self-esteem in children. |
    Compassion in children. | Resilience (Personality trait) in children. |
    Mindfulness (Psychology) | Emotions in children.
Classification: LCC BF575.S37 O43 2025 | DDC 155.4/124—dc23/eng/20240725
LC record available at https://lccn.loc.gov/2024016832

Contents

PART THREE

Tending Our Garden:
Integrating Self-Compassion into Family Life

Acknowledgments

We thank all the teachers, authors, and researchers who have inspired us on our path; those whom we have learned from along the way; individuals who have supported our practice of self-compassion and helped to inform our teaching and this book. We are particularly grateful for the work of the following authors and highly recommend you investigate their work as you explore self-compassion in the lives of your families: Christopher Germer, Kristin Neff, Shauna Shapiro, Tara Brach, Christopher Willard, Rick Hanson, Jack Kornfield, and James Baraz.

We would like to thank Thomas Masselis for his support and beautiful illustrations.

Louise would like to thank her friends and family and give special thanks to her mum, Margot, and dad, PJ. She would also like to thank David and her dear friends Isabell and Paul for their support and huge contribution to her work sharing mindfulness with children. Wendy would like to thank her incredibly supportive friends; her teacher, Chas; her husband, Dennis; and her children, Lauren and Ryan (both of whom also gave their permission to share some family stories).

Growing
Self-Compassionate
Children

Introduction

Welcome.

It is our heartfelt wish that within these pages you find support on the journey of self-compassion for yourself and the children in your life.

Based on our combined thirty-plus years of experience, we will share about self-compassion, its benefits, and how to practice this life-changing skill. From the foundation of your deepening understanding and practice, we will focus on accessible, practical, and fun ways to share these understandings and teachings with children. Though written with families in mind, all the practices and teachings shared here can be easily adapted in schools and other settings. Our intention is that this book may be of benefit anywhere there are children and adults who care for and about them. We passionately believe that supporting children in cultivating a kinder relationship with themselves and the world around them will help them bloom and develop resilience and capacity amid the challenges in life. Self-compassion can be a healing force for our children, families, communities, and world.

The book is organized into three sections. The first is focused primarily on the adult understanding of self-compassion and includes practical suggestions to develop this skill. The second is focused on sharing self-compassion with children, and the third is about integrating these practices more fully into family life. Though you may be tempted to skip over the section on self-compassion for adults, we encourage you not to do so. Self-compassion is, at its core, a way of relating to our experiences. For children to truly benefit, they need to see us, the adults in their lives, practice, embrace, and embody this way of being.

A message consistently echoed throughout this book is that your loving presence, supported by your practice, and your compassionate relationship with your child are essential to cultivating their self-compassion. The activities that you will find here are, as Louise likes to say, the icing on the cake, not the cake itself, and not substantial enough to stand on their own. Because everyone has different preferences and inclinations, there are multiple offerings. Please do not be overwhelmed by the number of options for the icing; simply try those that seem interesting to you and your family, and use them as they feel supportive.

The practices and teachings shared here are always offered as an invitation for both adults and children. As you work your way through the book, we encourage you to practice listening deeply to yourself and asking yourself, "What do I need?" If a practice doesn't feel right to you, trust your inner wisdom and skip it, or consider returning to it at another time. Be gentle with yourself and go at a pace that feels good to you, taking time to let the messages sink in and pausing for breaks as needed.

Finally, on a bit of a technical matter, although we collaborated on the entire book, we each took the lead on specific chapters in which we shared personal experiences. For ease of identification, we will include our name in parentheses the first time we express something from a personal perspective in each chapter. Please know that any other personal sharing in that chapter is from that individual.

With our best wishes that this book be of benefit to you and yours,

Wendy and Louise

If we take good care of ourselves, we help everyone. We stop being a source of suffering to the world, and we become a reservoir of joy and freshness.

—*Thich Nhat Hanh*

PART ONE

Preparing the Soil:
Self-Compassionate Adults

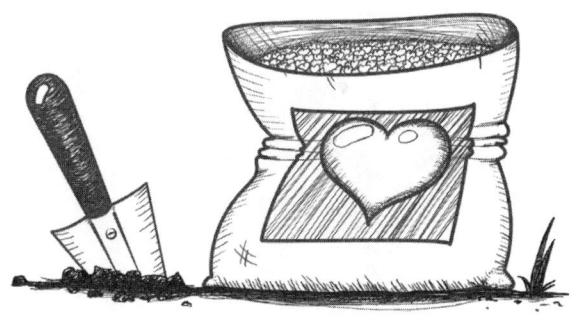

1

The Need for Self-Compassion in Our Lives

WE ALL WANT our children to be happy. This wish was clearly expressed by parents at a wellness workshop at my (Wendy's) children's school. Yet, as the facilitator adeptly pointed out, sometimes the ways we try to support their happiness can be counterproductive. Of course, there are many things we do and say that support our children's happiness. However, as was made apparent at the workshop, many of us also believe that in order for our children to be happy, we must also shield them from difficulties, including experiencing uncomfortable emotions. In this way, we don't see that a deeper sense of happiness comes not just from the pleasant experiences in life but also from our children having the ability and resilience to effectively handle life's inevitable stresses, challenges, and disappointments.

The truth is, sometimes things are difficult. Life doesn't always go our way. Things can be stressful and, at times, extremely challenging. Sometimes we don't get what we want or we get what we don't want. We all make mistakes, and regardless of the actual situation, many of us often feel we aren't good enough. Everyone feels hurt, worried, and insecure at times. This is true for adults and children. The better we understand this truth and develop the skills to manage those difficulties, the more at peace and truly happy we will be.

These struggles could be significant difficulties or just the countless disappointments or frustrations that happen as part of everyday life: things not going the way you want for yourself or your children. Often the most challenging situations are when we make a mistake or feel inadequate and experience harsh self-judgment or criticism. Whether it is significant life struggles, minor stressors, self-doubt, or criticism, they impact us daily, and how we relate to them makes a difference for ourselves and our children.

Consider if any of these have affected you or your child recently: a comment that hurt your feelings, having too much to do, saying something you were embarrassed about, not feeling included, technology issues, car problems, money stresses, work or school struggles, physical and mental health issues, or relationship difficulties. Like most of us, I have certainly experienced all of these and more. Regardless of our age, it is helpful to see that difficulties are a part of life and not add the additional burden of thinking that they mean that there is something wrong with us.

On some level, we know difficulties are a part of life, but how do we usually respond when things are hard? And is our response helpful? Is there a different way to relate to the challenges in life if we want to bloom fully, a way that could help fertilize the soil and make the flowers growing in our family garden a little more resilient? How can we best tend to this garden in difficult times and cultivate a more profound sense of well-being that comes from an ability to also be with the hard stuff, life's challenges, in a helpful way? After all, this is part of the human experience for each one of us.

There is growing evidence and reason to believe that self-compassion could do just that—that is, support our own well-being and our children's so we can bloom even amid adversity. We can learn to develop this resilience and stress hardiness for ourselves and teach it to our children.

You have picked up this book, so we suspect that helping your child manage life's challenges with grace, capacity, ease, and resilience is a priority. Understanding how people typically handle difficulties and why self-compassion may be beneficial will give you the foundation to do just that. You will be reminded throughout this book that your understanding, and especially your own practice of self-compassion, is the important first step. The adult's practice of self-compassion is the fertile soil that is needed to support a child in this way.

Before we delve more deeply, I want to be clear that I am not sharing anything here from the perspective of a parent who got it all, or even mostly, right. In fact, I made countless mistakes in the past and continue to do so. Parenting is wonderful and also really challenging at times. As my own self-compassion practice continues to develop, I am learning to give myself permission to be human and to be kinder to myself in those moments of difficulty. I tend to see my mistakes more quickly and clearly, make amends more easily as needed, and continue to learn and grow in my parenting and other areas of my life.

Our hope is that as you read along, you will see how developing your own self-compassion practice is a beautiful and helpful way to support yourself and your children on this journey. As was mentioned in the introduction, this part of the book will support you in working with difficulties in your life as well as specifically working with difficulties related to when your children struggle.

NOTICING THE WEEDS

There will be several opportunities for reflection throughout this book. If you like, consider using a journal to jot down your thoughts and feelings as a way to support you on this journey.

Think about the following questions as you begin to identify the particular weeds that can grow most often in your garden. It could be times you feel you have fallen short or made a mistake or the many ways that life can be challenging. As you get curious about the weeds that grow most often, you will be able to notice them more quickly and begin to proactively call on the resource of self-compassion to handle them more effectively. What are some of the weeds, life stressors, difficulties, and triggers for negative self-talk that keep you from fully blooming?

What didn't go my way today or this week?

What specific things tend to upset me or cause me distress?

What types of patterns do I notice in the things I tend to struggle with in my life right now? (Examples may be insecurities at work or worrying about my children.)

What things do I tend to be hard on myself about?

Handling the Weeds

When things are difficult, we make a mistake, or we feel we have "messed up" in some way, it can be beneficial to also pay attention to how we usually respond. I suggest approaching this and other opportunities for reflection in this book gently and with lots of kindness, especially when considering tendencies you feel may not be helpful for you or your family. Our intention is not to give ourselves a hard time about these habits but instead to develop a kind and interested curiosity to see more clearly what does and does not best support us. There is absolutely no judgment. Yet it is helpful to take the time to look closely, with interest and care, so we can begin to see where we may want to make some changes. Please do this with as much tenderness and understanding as possible as you navigate your way through this book.

Our Inner Critic

You may have noticed that little—or not so little—voice in your head that can say harsh and often hurtful things. In particular, it is not uncommon to turn on ourselves when we feel we haven't lived up to our own or others' expectations. This self-critical voice and even feelings of shame are companions for most of us at times. Though we may think they are sources of motivation, self-criticism and shame activate our threat defense response, releasing chemicals that inhibit the brain's learning centers. When our brain is affected in this way, we cannot learn and grow from our experiences.[1] Because shame is so painful, we are also hesitant to try new things or proactively approach challenges when the results of not being successful are so uncomfortable.

Whether or not we actually made a mistake, our minds often fall into the habit of self-criticism. You might take a moment to check in and see if this is true in your life. Do you ever find yourself lost in a story of not being as smart, kind, capable, talented, or good-looking as someone else? Of course, this list goes on, and the implication is that our value is determined by how we compare to others. Even without comparisons, we often believe we are not a good (or good enough) person, parent, partner, worker, friend, and so on. We can judge ourselves harshly or ruminate over something we did or said, worrying about how others might perceive us. The author and meditation teacher Tara Brach refers to this as "the trance of unworthiness," which is incredibly painful and, unfortunately, part of life for many of us as well as for our children.

As you reflect on the role of the inner critic in your life, you can also contemplate the impact it could have on your children. In particular, if you are outwardly harsh with yourself when you think you have made a mistake, consider if you may be giving your children the message that perfection is the expectation and that mistakes are unacceptable—a belief that so many of us have internalized from our childhood and from society. As you reflect on this, again, be sure to offer yourself lots of kindness for whatever you may notice.

When my children were young, I often found myself lost in thoughts about whether I was a good-enough parent, an experience I now realize is shared by so many others. My self-critic was incredibly loud and harsh in this area of my life, and further amplified by the fact that being a good mom was by far what was most important to me. I felt isolated with feelings of shame and doubt and was often caught up in painful stories of self-judgment. Over the years, mindfulness and self-compassion have been so helpful in this area of my life. I have learned ways to work with the inner critic including being kinder to myself when I am struggling in this way. This early parenting experience is why I have been so passionate about sharing these tools with other parents and am so grateful for the opportunity to share them with you here.

Ignore It and It Will Go Away

Another typical response to feeling like we made a mistake is covering over or avoiding looking at it. One way we do this is by pushing down the feelings and issues. But they do not go away; they wait, only to rise again, like a volcano. We may try to push down this sense of shame and discomfort by building up our self-esteem reserves and, conversely, putting down others. We blame others, as we haven't developed the capacity and support to look honestly and kindly at our mistakes. This keeps us from learning and growing from them.

Many of my friends are teachers. At the beginning of the school year, one message they try to impart to the students is that a mistake is an invitation to learn and grow. If our defenses are up and we are not willing to acknowledge our mistakes, we are destined to repeat them and will miss these important growth opportunities.

We also deal with challenging experiences in this way. We resist and avoid dealing with a difficulty directly or even acknowledging it exists. This resistance doesn't allow us to get close enough to work through whatever we are experiencing and can often lead to unhealthy coping strategies: scrolling the internet endlessly, eating a bag of chips without realizing it, consuming a few drinks, binge-watching TV, overspending, or even overworking. Insert your avoidance strategy here. What we resist persists; the more we try to push something away, the stronger we typically make it. Because this pattern of avoidance is below our conscious awareness, we are more likely to respond habitually and reactively or by using strategies that often increase harm and suffering.

The saying "Pain times resistance equals suffering," coined by the meditation teacher Shinzen Young, is apropos. We can't change the fact that there are difficulties in life (pain). When we relate to those difficulties with avoidance and resistance, we multiply our suffering. There will always be pain in life; however, with self-compassion, we can greatly reduce our suffering.

Overidentifying—Getting Lost in Our Emotions

When things are difficult, we can also respond by overidentifying with our feelings. We get caught up in our emotions and have no space to hold the difficulty. We can feel overwhelmed, as though the emotion is taking over. When this happens, our resilience is minimal, and we often feel the extra blame of "I can't handle things" or "Something is wrong with me." This reactive state of mind and heart is so uncomfortable and can leave us in even more emotional distress.

An analogy my meditation teacher, Chas DiCapua, has used is that of a storm. It can be overwhelming and all-consuming if we are outside in the middle of a raging storm. We can easily be reactive when caught in the storm of emotions. Our resilience is diminished. However, if we imagine looking at the storm from above, we can still see it, yet it doesn't have the same impact. We are aware of its presence and, from this vantage point, can even understand its origins and temporary nature, but we are not blown around by its intensity. From this more spacious perspective, we have an opportunity to choose how we respond.

HABITS FOR HANDLING
THE WEEDS REFLECTION

Knowing your habitual ways of reacting to life's ups and downs can be helpful as you begin to incline toward self-compassion. Once you know your usual responses, you can be on the lookout for them. They become a cue to stop and acknowledge that things are difficult and that this may be a good time to practice self-compassion.

With interest and kindness, ask yourself the following questions to begin to see more clearly how you relate to yourself in moments of difficulty. It may be helpful to journal using these questions as prompts.

What do I say to myself (silently or out loud), and what do I do when I have made a mistake?

When life is hard, how do I act, and what am I thinking and feeling at those times?

Do I get caught ruminating over past things I did or said? Do I spend a lot of time worrying about the future? How does it feel in my body and heart when I notice this?

Do I compare myself to others, and how does that feel?

Do I use any strategies mentioned in the chapter, such as ignoring or getting swept away or maybe harsh self-judgment? And if so, how does that feel?

What coping skills do I use—for example, overworking, food, and screen time?

What is my self-talk, and would I talk to a friend that way?

When things are hard, what impact does it have on my peace of mind, well-being, parenting, relationships, work, decisions . . .?

How Self-Compassion Can Help

In contrast, self-compassion gives us the tools to "be with" even the most challenging situations and emotions in a kind and loving way. It expands our ability to handle whatever arises, which helps us develop resilience. There is an implicit message in self-compassion about our inherent worth: simply because we exist, we, like all beings, are worthy of kindness and care when we are suffering.

Years ago, during an incredibly difficult family situation, a dear friend sent me an email that asked me to imagine she was wrapping me in a warm, soft, and comforting blanket. She said that the blanket was her love for me and to imagine I was being held in that love. She encouraged me to feel that blanket soothing me when things were hard as a way to soak in her love and support. Immediately I could feel her presence and deep care for me as I imagined being wrapped and held in this warm and comforting blanket. Using the analogy of the storm, self-compassion is the cozy blanket we can put on during the storm to soothe and comfort us.

With self-compassion as our companion, we have the courage to face the underlying issues and make changes to address them and heal as needed. Self-compassion makes it safe to make mistakes and comforts us if we believe the stories of our harsh inner critic, helping to soften its impact. It allows us to be with difficult experiences in life in a way that is kind and that cultivates strength and internal capacity.

Self-compassion has a physiological impact as it activates our caregiving system. Compassion is linked to oxytocin, the hormone that supports a sense of safety and connection. As we offer compassion to ourselves, it triggers the release of this hormone as well as endorphins, the feel-good neurotransmitters.[2] The impact of these chemicals ripples into our heart and mind, as they calm our nervous system and increase our capacity to effectively manage what arises from a place of safety and care.

Self-compassion is always available and is a reliable support in times of difficulty. We offer ourselves kindness because we are hurting; nothing else is required. An overview of the research on self-compassion shows a range of benefits. It is associated with happiness, higher levels of life satisfaction, and less depression and anxiety. The research on the many ways self-compassion benefits our well-being and resilience continues to grow.[3]

Understanding Self-Compassion

What exactly is self-compassion, and how can we begin to integrate it into our lives? I like to think of self-compassion as being a good friend to myself and believing that I truly deserve that care and kindness. Can I take the loving compassion I offer others and let that sunlight of care and kindness shine back on me? Can I offer myself some warmth and support in the midst of a difficult moment? Can I imagine wrapping myself in that cozy blanket of love and tenderness?

As was mentioned, these difficulties can be in terms of life's inherent stresses or when experiencing a difficult emotion or physical discomfort. It can also be when we are being hard on ourselves and feel we have fallen short in some way. Even in those moments when the self-critic is loud, can we still be caring toward ourselves, seeing that we are worthy of our kindness?

With self-compassion, we are holding our suffering and teaching children to hold theirs with affection. It can help to remember the intention of this practice, which is not to pretend that we didn't make a mistake or that everything is always perfect or to try to fix or change anything. It is simply to be kind to ourselves because we are hurting. We give ourselves compassion, not to get rid of feelings but because we feel bad. When a child falls and scrapes their knee, and we give them a kiss on the head, that kiss doesn't fix their knee, and yet, often, they do feel better. The act of kindness and care is, in itself, healing. Often we feel better simply because we feel cared for. This is a gift we can always offer ourselves, and I believe it is one of the greatest gifts we can share with our children.

> A moment of self-compassion can change your entire day. A string of such moments can change the course of your life.
>
> —*Christopher Germer*

In her research, self-compassion expert and author Kristin Neff describes self-compassion as having three components: mindfulness, common humanity, and self-kindness. We will delve more into these concepts in the following chapters. However, for our purposes, it is helpful to have a basic understanding to begin our exploration.

Mindfulness is an essential element in Neff's model of self-compassion. We must first see the difficulties and not be swept up in them or in denial for self-compassion to arise. I like to think of mindfulness as intentionally and wholeheartedly receiving each moment's experience with interest and kindness. It is the clarity and the warmth of the sun shining on whatever is happening now. Or, quite simply, as a meditation teacher shared during a retreat I attended: Here. Now. This.

With mindfulness, we are not fighting this moment's reality, which is essential for self-compassion. We must be willing to touch our suffering to then see it as a moment that could benefit from some kindness and care. When we get caught in the story, we need mindfulness to see that suffering is happening, especially when self-judgment is strong. As I criticize myself about something I said or did, can I pause and recognize that this is a moment of difficulty or that these feelings of self-judgment are painful? It is that clarity that is the power of mindfulness.

Neff's second aspect is common humanity. When things are not going as we would like, we tend to think something is wrong and take it personally. Though the particular situation and the degree of difficulty can vary greatly, it helps to remember that everyone struggles, makes mistakes, and feels bad about themselves and their lives sometimes. Seeing this shared reality as a part of being human helps to depersonalize emotions, decrease isolation, and keep us from adding another layer of self-judgment to an already difficult situation. It is, however, also important to note that common humanity isn't an attempt to minimize or dismiss our or our children's suffering. The tender and sincere acknowledgment of difficulty helps support us in truly seeing we are not alone when things feel hard.

Self-kindness, Neff's third aspect of self-compassion, is the ability to offer ourselves care and kindness during difficulties. It is a warm and authentic response to our challenges, whether external or in our minds. As we practice, we develop a loving and tender relationship with ourselves. When I am experiencing a challenging situation or struggling in my mind, I often ask myself, "Can I hold this with kindness?"

In the first wave of the coronavirus pandemic, I was on a Zoom call with a coalition of early education professionals. They were sharing about the enormous difficulties and struggles children and families were facing— problems many of these professionals with little ones of their own were also facing while trying to support others and adapt to the ever-changing landscape of the pandemic. They were exhausted, and the heaviness of the situation was quite palpable. At one point, someone in the group said in a kind and gentle tone, "This is just so hard." You could immediately feel a change in the group. It was like someone opened a release valve and let out some of the pressure. Everyone's face softened a bit, and the mood felt a little lighter. The acknowledgment of their shared suffering in a kind and warmhearted way hadn't changed the situation, but the validation, care, and shared support made such a difference.

Self-compassion can be a soothing way of speaking to ourselves, a gentle touch, or even a softening of the body. It can also be a more active or strength-based support, like setting boundaries or cheering ourselves on when things are hard. In those moments when I know a little bit of encouragement is what I need, I often say to myself, "This is hard, and I can handle it." Sometimes the strongest and most self-compassionate thing we can do is to acknowledge things are hard and to ask for help, something many of us find difficult and yet is such a crucial component of self-kindness.

During the Mindful Self-Compassion Teacher Training, I noticed a strong self-critical voice during one of the activities. Typically my response to this would be to offer myself some kind words and a soothing touch because my internal voice was harsh, and it was painful. However, this time I found myself saying, "This is an old story, and I don't need to believe you anymore." This protective, strong, motivating aspect of self-compassion is the focus of Neff's book *Fierce Self-Compassion* and is essential to our complete understanding of this practice.

Using Guided Practices

Throughout this book, there will be guided practices. If you would like to practice with your eyes closed, you can read through the instructions first and do the practice from memory. You can also periodically open your eyes to see the next instructions or even consider recording them. As with all the guided practices offered here, you are always encouraged to check in to see if you feel this practice is a good choice for you at this time.

This reminder about choice is important as we begin practicing self-compassion in the coming chapters. When we practice opening our hearts in the midst of our struggles, we can at times experience emotions more intensely. Know that it is not uncommon if offering yourself compassion is difficult at first or feels a bit overwhelming. If that happens, take a break. You could also consider using the Mindfulness of the Senses practice that will be covered in chapter 2 or feeling the sensations of your feet on the floor. Sometimes the most helpful thing to do is to use wise distraction, shifting your attention to doing something fun or physical.

SPRINKLING IN SOME SELF-COMPASSION

Now I invite you to try this brief practice, beginning to gently offer yourself some self-compassion. Like any new skill, it takes time and practice to develop. You can close your eyes if you like, and take a few gentle breaths to begin. Once you feel you have settled in, think of one challenging experience or a time you noticed a harsh inner critic. I suggest choosing something on the milder side, maybe a 4 or 5 on a scale of 1 to 10. It could be a minor disagreement with a partner or friend, feeling rushed in the mornings and being reactive, or second-guessing something you said or did.

As you recall the situation, notice where you were, what was happening, who was with you, and even the inner dialogue that may have taken place. Can you notice and even name the emotion you felt at that time? How does your body feel as you recall this situation?

Now gently invite your body to soften and your inner voice to be warm and soothing, then kindly ask yourself, "Can I hold this with kindness?"

Gently set the intention to invite the heart to open in the middle of this difficulty.

If it helps, you may tenderly place your hand on your heart as a reminder to be kind to yourself in this moment.

Notice how you feel now. How does your body feel? Your mind? Your heart? Know that however you feel is always okay. All your feelings are welcome.

With practice, you can begin to ask yourself this question and set this intention for self-kindness in the midst of a moment of difficulty, integrating self-compassion into your daily life.

QUESTIONS TO HELP US EXPLORE SELF-COMPASSION

We will pose the following four questions throughout the book:

How can I be with my difficulties?
How can I be with my child's difficulties?
How can I support my child in being with their difficulties?
How can I integrate self-compassion into family life?

Though many practices and activities will be included in the book, self-compassion is more than that. These practical tools and metaphors help train the heart, body, and mind to develop the habit of relating to ourselves with presence, love, and kindness. From the foundation of an authentic, embodied self-compassion practice, we can model and share this powerful skill and way of being with our children.

2

Practicing Kindness
toward Ourselves

I (LOUISE) LIKE TO describe mindfulness practice as shining a flashlight on our lives and ourselves; it is seeing both our inner and outer worlds more clearly. The author and meditation teacher Jon Kabat-Zinn describes mindfulness as "waking up to our lives." Yes, we do wake up to our lives, but this "waking up" can, at times, be a painful process. As we shine that flashlight of awareness on our internal world, often what we encounter is some level of discomfort and pain.

This was certainly the case in my own journey. After the initial honeymoon period with my mindfulness practice, I soon became more acutely aware of my pain and suffering. I could feel my body more, and as a result, I became more aware of its aches, pains, and uncomfortable sensations. I was also so much more aware of difficult thoughts and feelings, particularly thoughts of self-judgment. For me, those self-critical thoughts were quite relentless, and I realized my inner dialogue was often harsh and sometimes cruel. This was a painful realization. Although a core part of mindfulness practice is to relate to what we notice without judgment, I found it very difficult to simply "be" with my own pain. I have since discovered that many others have similar experiences on their own journeys with mindfulness practice.

A major turning point came when I first encountered Kristin Neff's work on mindful self-compassion. As I read Neff's words and listened to her talks and meditations, I realized that although I was strongly motivated to relate to others with kindness and compassion, this was something that I rarely offered myself. Inspired by the work of the psychologist and mindfulness expert Shauna Shapiro, I began to bring a quality of kindness to my attention by infusing my attention with kindness—in both my meditation practice and everyday life. Although I was still encountering uncomfortable thoughts, feelings, and sensations, this healing balm of kindness supported me to be with these difficulties, and, in turn, my suffering began to ease. I felt more at peace and content in my life. I also noticed that as my self-kindness developed, my ability to offer genuine care and kindness to others also deepened.

I am certainly not alone in my struggle with self-judgment. Throughout my years working as a mindfulness teacher, I have discovered that frequently our deepest struggle as human beings is not other people or external difficulties but rather with the turbulent, often painful relationships we have with our own selves.

> I believe that the sense of not being enough is the most pervasive suffering in our society.
>
> —*Tara Brach*

So many of us would never dream of speaking to or treating others the way we relate to ourselves. It is almost like, at times, we disregard our own humanity. Parents, in particular, can become burdened by thoughts of inadequacy and harsh self-judgment.

Drawing on personal experience and my work with others, we will consider the first question posed at the beginning of the book: "How can I be with my difficulties?" One of the most transformational steps we can take to support our own well-being is to begin the journey of befriending our lives and ourselves. I believe that the relationship that we have with who we are is our most important relationship—after all, we are always with ourselves. We can be surrounded by loving partners, children, family, and friends, but if we are essentially in deep conflict with who we are, then we are likely to experience considerable suffering.

I also believe that we genuinely have a choice regarding the quality of the relationship we have with ourselves. We can spend our lives comparing ourselves to others, judging our bodies, and putting ourselves down, or we can make the choice to begin befriending and making peace with ourselves. Through the cultivation of mindfulness and compassion practices, we can begin to bring a "loving acceptance" to the people we are, the bodies we have, the lives we live, and even to our pain and struggles. We can turn toward our beautiful, human, perfectly imperfect selves with presence, gentleness, love, and care.

When we foster genuine kindness and compassion for ourselves, we will look after ourselves well. We will care for our minds, hearts, and bodies. We will be less likely to put ourselves in danger or to do anything that might harm ourselves or others.

In addition, our relationship with ourselves sets the tone for every other relationship in our lives. If we have cultivated a loving, caring relationship with ourselves, our relationships with others will tend to reflect this.

If your compassion does not include yourself, it is not complete.

—*Jack Kornfield*

Self-compassion can act like a healing, comforting balm that soothes us through the difficult moments of our lives. Parenting is such a demanding job, and although I am not a parent myself, I have worked with hundreds of parents throughout my career. I have witnessed so many parents battle with themselves, judging themselves and their parenting so harshly. I think the line from the poem "Bapuji Says" by Swami Kripalvananda demonstrates the impact of this judgment so well: "Each time we judge ourselves, we break our own hearts."

Although we might not realize it at the time, we actually break our own hearts when we treat ourselves so harshly, and this does have an impact on our happiness and well-being. Life already has plenty of difficulties, and parenting, while bringing great joy and fulfillment, also comes with many challenges. Wouldn't it be wonderful if we approached parenting as a period in our lives to really focus on wrapping ourselves in that "warm blanket of self-compassion," a time to give ourselves more compassion, not less; more gentleness, kindness, and care, not less?

We Cannot Give What We Do Not Have

One of the most important benefits of befriending ourselves is that once we are genuinely practicing kindness and compassion for ourselves, we will also be authentically modeling this for our children. Many of the parents I work with are very motivated to teach their children about self-kindness and self-compassion. Parents are often eager to learn specific techniques and activities that they can share with their children. While this is wonderful, the reality is that many of these parents struggle themselves with harsh self-criticism and self-judgment.

If we want to encourage self-compassion in our children, the most important thing we can do as parents and caregivers is to genuinely embody a loving, caring relationship with ourselves. Children will learn so much more about self-compassion by experiencing this authentically modeled by a parent than from any technique or activity we might present to them. So, if we truly want to support our children to be self-compassionate, then we need to begin the journey of embodying this in our own bodies, minds, and hearts.

I like to use the "cup" analogy to demonstrate this embodiment of self-compassion. Imagine we have a cup. In this cup is what we have to give our children. Imagine we have tea in our cup. We might really want to give our children milk, for example. We might read lots of books about milk and know that milk is really good for our children, but if we only have tea in our cup, then all we can give them is tea, no matter how much we want to give them milk. We cannot give what we do not have! If we want to give our children the gift of self-compassion, then the very best thing we can do is to fill up our own cups with compassion and kindness for ourselves.

Reading about self-compassion and having an intellectual understanding of the concept can be helpful, but what actually fills our cup is the consistent practice of self-compassion. We can think of this as a bit like learning to play the piano. We can read every book in the world about playing the piano, and we can even write a doctoral thesis on playing the piano, but we will never fully understand what it means to play the piano until we actually play it. In the same way, we do not know how to play the piano after practicing it only once or twice. We need to play the piano again and again and again. Beginning our journey toward embodying self-compassion is just like this. We need to practice it repeatedly, ideally as a daily practice. In the words of Shauna Shapiro, "What we practice grows stronger." If you truly want to cultivate self-compassion, the most helpful advice I could give you is to keep practicing and to integrate self-compassion as a way of being into your everyday life to the best of your ability.

In addition, if we wanted our child to learn how to play the piano, we would not send them to a teacher who has only read about playing the piano or who has only practiced the piano a few times. We would send them to a teacher who is a competent piano player. It is the same thing with self-compassion. As a parent, you are your child's greatest teacher. They are observing you and learning from you all the time. As you develop your practice of self-compassion, your child will be learning to be kind to themselves by simply being in your presence. As you treat yourself and speak to yourself with kindness, your child will learn to relate to themself in a similar way.

How Can We Cultivate Self-Kindness?

There are two main ways that we can practice self-compassion: formally and informally. We can practice self-compassion informally by simply bringing a kind, compassionate attitude to ourselves as we go throughout our day, particularly when we encounter moments of difficulty or suffering. Formal practice involves explicitly practicing specific self-compassion-based meditations and reflections. Many of these formal and informal practices are included throughout this book. The main difference is that when we practice formally, we make time specifically for that practice and do not do anything else—for example, practicing a five-minute self-compassion-based meditation, sitting with eyes closed. In informal practice, we simply go about our day as we normally would while at the same time relating to ourselves with self-compassion—for example, speaking kindly to ourselves and putting a hand on our heart during a moment when we are struggling while our child is having a tantrum.

As mentioned in the previous chapter, Kristin Neff has outlined three components of self-compassion: mindfulness, common humanity, and kindness. When we fill our own cups with these components, then we will be able to model self-compassion to our children authentically. We will be able to give our children what is genuinely in our cup, and we will experience the benefits that self-compassion practice can bring to our own lives. The section below will delve more deeply into the three components of self-compassion with some practices that will help us begin or continue on our journey.

Mindfulness

If self-compassion can be thought of as bringing kindness to our suffering, then in order to do this, we first must have a conscious awareness that we are experiencing some kind of discomfort. As mentioned previously, we can think of mindfulness like a flashlight. It allows us to bring more awareness or "light" to what is happening in our internal and external worlds.

I like to describe mindfulness as paying attention to what is happening as it is happening, without judgment and with kindness. A helpful way to view mindfulness is as a practice and as a way of "being" rather than a destination to reach or a theoretical concept.

Mindfulness is something that needs to be experienced to be fully understood, just as to fully comprehend what it means to drive a car, we have to actually drive the car and do so repeatedly. Reading books about driving cars will only give us a very limited level of understanding. Reading about mindfulness is, of course, helpful, but it is the practice of mindfulness that is most important. Mindfulness is also very much like a muscle—the more we exercise our muscle of mindfulness, the stronger it becomes; and like a muscle, we must maintain our practice to keep it strong.

The following section includes practices to support you in strengthening your mindfulness muscle. Mindfulness works best if we incorporate it into our lives as a daily practice. However, it is important not to judge or criticize yourself if you struggle with or forget to do the practices. Although the concept of mindfulness seems quite straightforward, the practice itself can be challenging. I suggest making an intention to simply try your best to follow the recommendations here. Each time we practice mindfulness, we can celebrate and congratulate ourselves. When we struggle or forget to practice, we can remember that this is very normal and relate to ourselves with kindness and care rather than judgment or criticism.

MINDFULNESS OF THE SENSES

When we bring our attention to what is happening in the present moment, noticing the information that we receive from our five senses, we are practicing mindfulness. Throughout the day, practice bringing your attention to your five senses. Simply notice what you can see, hear, smell, taste, and touch in that particular moment. It can also work well to practice Mindfulness of the Senses in nature—going for a mindful walk, for example, noticing the feeling of the sun on your skin, the sounds of the birds tweeting, or the colors of the trees. Another wonderful way to practice "mindful senses" is when we are spending time with our child. We can simply be with our child, noticing the sound of their voice, the smell of their skin, the touch of their hands, and the sight of their beautiful smile.

MINDFUL BREATHING

Our breathing is always happening in the "now." A great way to practice mindfulness is simply to bring awareness to your breath in any particular moment. You don't have to change your breathing in any way. You can simply notice the feeling of your breath moving through your body. Ask yourself, "How does it feel to breathe in this moment?" As you breathe in, be aware that you are breathing in, and as you breathe out, be aware that you are breathing out. You can also practice saying the words "Here" as you breathe in and "Now" as you breathe out.

Mindfulness can also be practiced as a formal sitting practice. To begin, set a timer on your phone for the length of time that you would like to practice. You can start off with a short period of practice; even one minute is perfect. I suggest a seated posture, sitting tall like a mountain, keeping your back straight; softening the muscles in your face, shoulders, and belly; and, if you like, closing your eyes. Now begin to bring your awareness to your breath. As you breathe, focus on the feeling of the breath in your body—your tummy moving or the sensation of air entering or leaving your nostrils. Alternatively, you can simply notice the overall feeling of your body breathing. Feel the breath moving like waves through your body. Allow your breathing to bring you home to yourself and the present moment.

When your mind wanders away from the breath to a thought, notice that thought with kindness and without judgment, then bring your attention back to your breath. Remember, you are not trying to stop your mind from thinking; it is the nature of the mind to think in the same way as it is the nature of the heart to beat. You are simply noticing when you are thinking and then gently and kindly bringing your focus back to your breathing. As you get more used to the practice, you can increase the length of time.

LABELING THOUGHTS AND EMOTIONS

As we develop our mindfulness practice, we become more aware of what is happening in our internal world. We become more aware of our thoughts, feelings, and bodily sensations. A really supportive way to relate to what is happening within us is to practice the labeling technique. Labeling helps us to create more space around our thoughts and feelings, seeing them more clearly and being less identified with them. It can also help reduce the amount of reactivity we experience around our inner experience. You can begin the labeling practice with thoughts initially.

In both your informal and formal mindfulness practice, you will notice that your mind frequently wanders away from the present moment into thoughts. Try bringing awareness to what type of thought you are thinking and gently label it, then return to your breathing. If you were practicing mindful breathing, for example, and you noticed that you were thinking about a conversation with your child's teacher yesterday, you would label the thought as "past thought," then let it go without judging it and connect back to the present moment through your breath.

You can deepen this practice by also labeling emotions. As you go throughout your day, pause and bring your attention to your body with the same attitude of kindness and curiosity that you would give to a really dear friend. Now ask yourself, "What emotion or emotions am I feeling at this moment?" Sometimes you will notice that you are feeling more than one emotion. Practice labeling the emotion or emotions that are present by gently saying the name of the emotion to yourself using a soft, soothing tone—for example, "fear, fear . . . ," or you could say, "This is fear." Try not to judge whatever emotion or emotions you experience as you practice.

NOTICING MOMENTS OF SUFFERING

As we start to shine the flashlight of mindfulness on ourselves and our lives, we begin to notice more of everything: comfortable, pleasurable experiences; neutral experiences; and moments of discomfort and suffering. This is an important step in order to be able to authentically offer ourselves self-compassion, as we need to be aware that we are suffering in order to bring kindness and compassion to the discomfort we are experiencing. In this practice, we are noticing and labeling difficult or uncomfortable moments.

When you are experiencing a moment of difficulty or discomfort, try pausing and taking a breath, gently bringing your attention to your body, and see if you can notice and label the feeling you're experiencing.

Begin by describing to yourself the situation that you are in. For example, if the kids are fighting and you are feeling stressed, you could softly say to yourself:

The kids are fighting today.
I am feeling stressed.

Then you can affirm to yourself that this is a difficult moment, that this is a moment of suffering. In a tender, soothing voice, you could say to yourself:

I am suffering in this moment.
This is hard.
I am finding this moment difficult.
I am struggling right now.

It is helpful to practice with different phrases to find what particular words feel most supportive for you.

Common Humanity Practice

Kristin Neff describes self-compassion as "loving, connected presence." While mindfulness helps us cultivate presence, "common humanity" helps us cultivate a sense of being connected to others. Common humanity gives us the understanding that we are not alone in our suffering, that difficulties and suffering are part of life and certainly part of being a parent. Through common humanity, we understand that we are not the only ones struggling or finding life difficult.

I AM NOT THE ONLY ONE

When you are aware that you are struggling or having a difficult moment, pause, take a breath, and say to yourself, "And I am not the only one." So, for example, after having an argument with your partner and you feel frustrated and upset, try pausing and saying to yourself in a gentle, soothing tone, "This is difficult and upsetting, and I am not the only one." Or perhaps you are having a hard time getting the baby to sleep, and you are exhausted and overwhelmed. Pause, take a deep breath, and say to yourself, "I am absolutely exhausted, and I am not the only one."

You can experiment with other phrases that help connect you to a sense of common humanity during moments of struggle or difficulty. Examples of phrases that might be helpful include:

There are so many others who are feeling just like me right now.
Parenting is difficult for everyone at times.
Suffering is part of the human experience; I am not alone in feeling like this.
There are so many other parents in a similar situation.
Feeling like this is a part of being human.

The most important thing is that the phrases feel supportive to you and help you feel connected to others during moments of difficulty.

Practicing Kindness toward Ourselves

One of the greatest gifts we can give ourselves is the gift of making friends with who we are. We are always with ourselves, and we always have ourselves. When we begin to embody a kind, loving inner voice, the struggles and the suffering we experience in life can be soothed and eased.

We can begin our "self-kindness" practice by meeting ourselves exactly where we are at this moment. Wherever we are starting from is always absolutely okay. The following practices may assist you in beginning to gently cultivate a kinder, more loving relationship with yourself. These practices are especially helpful in supporting us to be with our difficulties.

INTENTION FOR SELF-KINDNESS

Practicing with "intention" can help us turn the compass of our hearts toward relating to ourselves with more kindness and care in our daily lives. We can begin the day with the intention to be kind. You might like to write your intention down first thing in the morning or write colorful intentions on heavy paper or stones and pop them around the house or in your pocket or handbag as a reminder for yourself. Practice finding words that feel like a good "fit" for you. Examples of "kind intentions" might include:

> May I be kind to myself today.
> May I honor and value myself today.
> May I be a friend to myself today.
> May I nurture and nourish myself today.
> May I love and accept myself today.
> May I protect and provide for myself today.
> May I give myself what I need today.

We can pause throughout the day and come back to our intention, noticing if we are relating to ourselves in accordance with our intention and reorienting ourselves toward it if needed. Remember that every moment is a perfect chance to start again.

BEING OUR OWN BEST FRIEND

As was mentioned in chapter 1, one of the most effective ways of cultivating "self-kindness" is to practice relating to ourselves in the same way we would relate to our most dear and precious friend. When we are experiencing a moment of difficulty, we can ask ourselves, "How would I relate to a friend in a similar situation? What would my attitude toward my friend be? What words might I offer my friend? What tone of voice would I use when I speak to them?" We can then begin caring for ourselves in a similar way.

We can notice the attitude we are bringing toward ourselves. What is the quality of our attention? Are we judging ourselves, comparing ourselves to others, telling ourselves that something is not okay, that we are falling short or lacking in some way? Then we can begin to infuse our attention with gentleness and kindness, relating to ourselves the way we would relate to someone we dearly love. We can notice our "self-talk," the words we are saying to ourselves, and explore if we can speak to ourselves in a gentler, kinder way.

KIND TOUCH

The Mindful Self-Compassion program, developed by Christopher Germer and Kristin Neff, highlights the importance of "soothing touch." Offering ourselves "kind touch" is a beautiful way to relate to ourselves with kindness and compassion. When we notice we are experiencing a moment of struggle or difficulty, we can care for ourselves well by giving ourselves the same sort of gentle touch that we might offer our child or a dear friend.

We can imagine our hands are filled with kindness and compassion, and we can picture this streaming through our fingers toward ourselves. We can experiment with what type of touch feels best and most soothing for us.

Helpful practices include:

Putting a hand or both hands on our heart.
Putting one hand on our heart and one hand on our tummy.
Gently holding our tummy with both hands.
Putting one hand in a fist on your heart and the other placed over the fist.
Putting a hand on our cheek.

Putting both hands on our cheeks, gently holding our face.

Holding our hands or gently squeezing our hands.

Hugging or gently squeezing ourselves.

Putting both hands on our forehead.

Putting one hand on our forehead and one hand at the top or base of our head.

We can experiment with the type of touch that feels best and is most soothing for us. This may differ from day to day and be based on the type of difficulty we are going through.

WHAT DO I NEED?

This is one of my favorite practices, and I feel that when we consistently bring this into our lives, it can be quite transformational. At any moment, we can pause, take a breath, and ask ourselves, "What is it that I most need at this moment?" Deeply listen to yourself and ask yourself what it is that would most support you in that moment. Then gently ask yourself, "How can I give myself what it is that I need?"

This practice is particularly helpful when we are experiencing moments of unease and difficulty.

We can expand this practice by putting a hand gently on our forehead. We can ask, "What does my mind need?" We can then put one hand on our heart and one hand on our tummy and ask ourselves, "What does my body need?" We can put two hands on our heart and ask ourselves, "What does my heart need?"

Bring loving awareness to your being, to your body, mind, and heart, truly listening to yourself with curiosity and kindness. Sometimes you might discover that you need to bring a certain quality to yourself; you might need to offer yourself more acceptance or forgiveness, for example. Other times, you might find that what best supports you is a kind action, such as going out for a walk, having a cup of tea, asking for help, or speaking to a friend. On occasion, what is most needed may be setting a clear boundary with a person or situation.

The meditation teacher and author James Baraz suggests making a "nourishment list" of the people, experiences, and material objects in your life that nourish you and bring you joy. You can then try integrating the items on your nourishment list into your life whenever you can.

THE SELF-COMPASSION BREAK

We can bring the practices outlined above together using an exercise from the Mindful Self-Compassion program called the Self-Compassion Break. The Self-Compassion Break can be practiced any time you notice that you are struggling or suffering in some way. We can practice the Self-Compassion Break informally as we go throughout our day by following the steps outlined below.

There are three main steps to the Self-Compassion Break, which incorporate the three components of self-compassion: mindfulness, common humanity, and self-kindness.

STEP 1: NOTICE THAT YOU ARE SUFFERING

During moments when we are experiencing difficulty, we can pause, take a deep breath, and affirm to ourselves that "this is a difficult moment" or "this is a moment of suffering." You can also use the other phrases suggested in the Noticing Moments of Suffering practice mentioned earlier in this chapter.

STEP 2: CONNECT TO OUR COMMON HUMANITY

The next step is to connect to a sense of common humanity. You can say to yourself, "I am not the only one who is in a situation like this. There are many others who are feeling this way right now. Feeling this way is part of being human." Again, you can also experiment with the phrases suggested in the I Am Not the Only One practice in this chapter.

STEP 3: TURN TOWARD YOURSELF WITH KINDNESS

We can then begin to bring an attitude of "self-kindness" toward ourselves. Ask yourself the question, "How would I treat a good friend in the same situation?" Now practice relating to yourself in the same way that you would treat a good friend who was going through something similar. Try speaking to yourself with kind words and offer yourself soothing touch. Perhaps engage in a "kind action" that might support you, asking yourself, "What do I most need in this moment?"

Other supportive prompts may include "What do I most need to hear in this moment?" or "What would allow my heart to rest, at least a little?" We can also ask ourselves, "Do I need help right now?" and perhaps ask for support from others when appropriate. The exercises described in the previous section, "Practicing Kindness toward Ourselves," may also be supportive for you here. The most important thing is that the words, phrases, gestures, and prompts you offer yourself feel like a good fit for you. Practice listening to your body, trusting its wisdom and experimenting with what most brings a sense of ease and comfort during moments of difficulty. I like to describe this practice as "listen, listen, listen, love, love, love."

You can also practice the Self-Compassion Break formally by taking a few minutes to reflect on a situation that you are finding difficult at the moment and then applying the three steps outlined above to the situation and how it is impacting you. You can try this with eyes open or closed, whichever you find most comfortable. You might also like to take some time to journal, reflecting on any insights you may have received.

Misconceptions of Self-Compassion

Pause, take a nice deep breath, and take some time to reflect on the following questions, perhaps in a journal: How is it for you when you consider the possibility of being kinder and more compassionate to yourself? Do you notice that you feel any blocks or resistance to practicing self-compassion? What are some thoughts or beliefs that may hinder your practice of self-compassion?

Remember, there are no right or wrong answers to these questions. We can simply bring awareness and nonjudgment to any insights we might have. We can hold anything we might notice in kind, compassionate attention.

In my work sharing these practices with others, I have noticed that some people can experience resistance to practicing self-compassion due to feeling that it may be self-indulgent or selfish. Others think it will make them lazy or unproductive, and some may view self-compassion as weak or narcissistic. In fact, a growing body of research on the impact of self-compassion practice indicates that these perceptions are false.

Research demonstrates that self-compassion practice is a source of inner strength that supports courage and promotes resilience when we're faced with difficulties. Self-compassion supports long-term health and well-being rather than short-term pleasure, with self-compassionate people tending to engage in healthier behaviors like exercising, eating well, and drinking less. Rather than being lazy or unproductive, self-compassionate people have high personal standards. However, they don't harshly judge themselves when they make mistakes or fail. Self-compassionate people genuinely care about themselves and want to reach their full potential and goals in life.[4]

Personally I feel that cultivating self-compassion is one of the kindest things we can do for the people in our lives, especially our children. As we fill up our own cup with self-compassion, we have better mental and physical health, we are more rested, we have more energy, and we certainly have a greater capacity to care for our loved ones. Also, as we meet our own precious, "messy" human selves in a kind, loving, nonjudgmental way, we develop a greater capacity to meet our children and others in our lives in a similar way. Wouldn't it be beautiful to view our self-compassion practice as an act of kindness not only for ourselves but also for every other human being whom we encounter in our lives?

3

Supporting Ourselves When Our Children Are Struggling

Here we will begin to delve into the second question posed at the beginning of the book: "How can I be with my child's difficulties?" Keeping in mind that self-compassion for parents could be a book in itself, our focus will be on those areas that most relate to this question.

A North Star for Relating to Our Children

During an interview, as he was discussing training mindful self-compassion teachers, Steve Hickman, former executive director of the Center for Mindful Self-Compassion, said that to teach it, you must practice it. He used the phrase previously mentioned and commonly used in the Mindful Self-Compassion program: "to be a loving, connected presence." More than any explicit sharing of tools or strategies, the teacher's capacity to truly embody this way of relating to experiences, especially the unpleasant ones, enables us to teach it authentically to others. The same holds true in our role as parents. For mindful self-compassion teachers and for us as parents, this is an ongoing process, not an ideal to achieve but a North Star in our lives, an intention or directionality.

Though I (Wendy) have been practicing mindfulness and self-compassion for many years, and my children are now adults, my radar is still on high alert for times when they may be struggling. My desire for their happiness and well-being remains a strong and powerful force in my life. This force, and many old habits, can get in the way of this intention: to be a loving, connected presence in my own life and in theirs. At times, I still catch myself responding to their difficulties in ways that are unhelpful to us all, trying to fix or minimize the situation and emotions, or just getting caught in the story.

I share this as an important reminder. This chapter—in fact, this book—isn't about perfecting yourself as a parent. Instead, we hope to point to a way of embracing all the messiness of parenting more fully and with as much love and kindness as possible.

As my self-compassion practice has deepened, I have come to view my parenting as an ongoing learning process with new opportunities to fall down and get back up around every corner. Remembering that "falling down" is an essential and normal part of the process has helped me offer myself much-needed self-kindness when I feel I haven't lived up to my parenting expectations.

In the previous chapter, we looked at setting an intention for self-kindness in general. Now, as we look at setting intentions around how we want to show up for our children, I encourage you to hold these intentions gently and with as much care and curiosity as possible. When you feel you have not parented as you would have hoped, can you be interested in what got in the way and what can be learned while holding yourself with deep kindness? When my children were young, I read many parenting books and often felt some underlying judgment, pressure, or expectation to have it all together. I could never live up to the ideal put forward. Please know there are no ideals here, just gentle encouragement to set an intention and then be interested and kind to yourself with whatever arises.

We set an intention because there is power in pointing ourselves in a particular direction as parents, even if we can get a bit off course sometimes. We are inclining the mind to do it differently. Our habits are strong, and to make a change requires a level of intentionality, a purposeful shift of the mind in that direction. A clear intention helps us look for opportunities to use and practice these new tools and skills. It can be as simple as setting an intention to offer ourselves comfort and care in the midst of our child's difficulty and to support our child as they learn to hold their struggles in a kind and caring way.

SETTING YOUR PARENTING NORTH STAR

The Setting Your Parenting North Star practice takes the intention-setting activity from the previous chapter one step further, with a focus on how you want to show up for your child, especially amid difficulties.

It may be helpful to have a journal or some paper nearby for the reflection component of this activity. Close your eyes if you like, and take a few gentle breaths. Bring to mind a time as a child when you were mildly hurt—maybe a scraped elbow or a minor experience of hurt feelings. On a scale of 1 to 10, try to come up with something that is in the 4 or 5 range.

Allow yourself to remember and feel what it was like to have that experience. Now imagine an adult coming over and caring for you, giving you a hug or a kiss on the head, if that is comfortable for you, or being deeply present for you in some way that feels kind and supportive. This could be a real person who, for you, embodies kindness and compassion or an imaginary being offering tenderness and care. As you imagine this experience, notice how it feels emotionally as well as in your body to be so lovingly cared for in a moment of difficulty. How does it feel to be with this individual who is offering you care?

Circle or write down any of the following words that relate to your experience with this person: *trust, love, acceptance, presence, authenticity, receptivity, attunement, connection, spaciousness, held, comforted, seen, empowered, interested, gentle, kind, open, tender, soft.* You can also add your own words here.

Now, with this embodied reminder of compassionate presence and some words to draw on, set an intention for how you would like to show up for yourself and your child in those moments of hurt, disappointment, or difficulty. It could be something like "to be a gentle and accepting presence" or another phrase that resonates with you. As was mentioned in the previous chapter, you can also put this intention on paper, decorate a rock with the words, or even write it on a sticky note so you can refer to it periodically. Possibly place it in a location where you will see it first thing in the morning to start your day with a reminder of your intention.

Starting with Ourselves

To truly understand how to support our children when they are having a hard time, we must first recognize how intimately connected we are to their internal experiences. We are deeply affected when someone we love is struggling, especially our children. This is why it is essential to practice being with our inner experience before relating to our children in moments of difficulty. How do we relate to ourselves in those moments when our child is disappointed, hurt, or struggling in some way? As we come to see and understand our habitual reactions, we can develop the ability to work with them more effectively. This capacity for working with our own feelings is what is needed to best support our children with their difficult experiences and emotions. Connecting first with our own hearts, bodies, and minds before reaching out to relate to theirs.

In private sessions with parents and children, I often saw just how deeply our children's struggles impact us, the adults who love and care for them. I can still remember how painful it was for one mom as she shared about her child being the only one in his "friend" group not invited, yet again, to a party. She was heartbroken for her son and worried about his ongoing well-being. Her child's experience—like so many of us who have experienced a time when our child was left out, lonely, or felt they didn't belong—had affected her deeply. The fact is, it hurts when our child is suffering.

This is the moment to check in with ourselves. Can we be with our uncomfortable feelings first so we can better help our children be with theirs? To offer self-compassion, we must acknowledge these unpleasant feelings in order to hold them lovingly. It takes practice and intention to not instinctively try to get rid of, fix, or ignore uncomfortable feelings, so be patient as you move in this direction. When we are unable to be with the discomfort and unpleasantness of our own and our children's tricky emotions, the inclination is to use coping skills that, though well intended, aren't typically helpful.

STOP AND TAKE A BREATH

One way to practice slowing down so we can check in with ourselves when our child is dealing with difficulties is to stop and take a breath. In *Breathing Makes It Better*, the children's book I coauthored with Christopher Willard, it repeatedly says, "Stop and take a breath." This is a helpful instruction for adults as well as children. When someone we love hurts, our reactivity can make it hard to respond effectively. At moments like this, the first step can simply be to stop and breathe. A little pause to take even one conscious breath before responding can make a tremendous difference.

Contrary to what our fast-paced society might have us believe, most things do not usually require an immediate response, even an emotionally struggling child. Typically, you and your loved ones will benefit if you stop and breathe. Pausing in this way gives you the gift of a little time to calm your nervous system. You will be less likely to be reactive and have a bit more choice in how you respond.

Comparing, Self-Judgment, and Shame

We previously discussed our inner critic as one way many of us respond internally when things are hard—a way that deepens our suffering and could greatly benefit from some self-compassion. This is especially true when our child is having a hard time, because harsh self-judgment, comparing, and shame impact our ability to take care of our emotions and support our children most effectively. These difficult internal experiences are powerful influences in many of our lives. Here, we will investigate these topics further, specifically as they relate to times when our child is struggling, and learn some self-compassionate responses that can help minimize their impact on us.

Yes, the mother on social media does seem to have it all together, and there are countless ways we get the message that a perfect family is an attainable goal. Of course, we know consciously that what we see on social media is not the whole picture and often not even close to the accurate picture, and yet those images still influence us. Remember, no one out there is getting it "right"—not the person on social media or the parent at your child's school who always appears to be doing it all perfectly. We are all just human beings learning and growing and doing our best. A kind reminder here is to limit exposure to these sources if they are making you feel inadequate. Notice how your body, heart, and mind feel when reading a blog or looking at someone's social media and decide if this is someone whose advice or presence in your life is beneficial to you. You can ask yourself if this is helping or harming you or if it is supporting you in treating yourself with kindness and care.

If your child is having a hard time, it is common to look around and think you are the only one whose child is struggling and to judge yourself and your parenting. As parents, we often set unrealistic expectations for ourselves and our children. Being truly present with our child's difficulties can be even more challenging when this happens. This is where the reminder about common humanity is so important. Every family, every child, every parent, every caregiver—in fact, every person—struggles sometimes. They just don't put it on social media. Every child has meltdowns and particular things that are hard for them: school difficulties, sensory struggles, worry, feelings of overwhelm, and friendship problems, to name a few.

When my son was in middle school and it became apparent that he was having some difficulties, I began hearing from other mothers in his friend group. At first I thought they wanted to be "supportive," which often meant giving advice and talking about their children's achievements. Instead, now that the door was open, many were quietly looking for support and resources to help their own children. Though I had no idea and, in fact, assumed things were going perfectly for them, many of these children and parents were also having a hard time.

Once we are willing to be vulnerable and share our parenting struggles, other parents often feel safe to do the same. It is incredibly helpful to find people you can trust who are willing and able to be real and genuine about parenting. I know from personal experience what a difference it can make to have authentic relationships with other parents based on kindness, honesty, and compassion. All parents and children experience hard times. When we fail to see this, we easily fall into the trap of harsh self-judgment.

Self-judgment can quickly turn into shame, where we not only feel bad about what happened but perceive ourselves as bad, unworthy, or unacceptable in some way, particularly in our role as parents. Because shame grows in isolation, a reminder of common humanity and kindness can be beneficial when you feel you are headed into the quicksand of shame.

In her book *The Magnanimous Heart: Compassion and Love, Loss and Grief, Joy and Liberation*, Narayan Helen Liebenson tells the story of being initially surprised when a meditation teacher said to her, "You will make many mistakes." I find such freedom in this statement and wish someone had said it to me as a young parent. Accepting the truth of our humanity, that it is impossible not to make mistakes, even—or especially—in the realm of parenting, helps open the door to learning from them.

To be human is to be imperfect.

—*Kristin Neff*

The following practices can be particularly supportive for working with self-judgment and shame.

JUST LIKE ME, HOW HUMAN OF ME

Just like you, everyone, including every child, will experience difficulties. We increase our suffering in those moments when we feel isolated, as though no one else is experiencing these struggles. So often we may wonder,

"What is wrong with me? What is wrong with my parenting? What is wrong with my child?" Wanting our children to be happy is part of the parent job description. All parents want their children to be happy, and all parents experience the heartache that comes when their child is having a hard time. Similar to the I Am Not the Only One practice in the previous chapter, when we feel isolated or some self-judgment in relation to our parenting or our child's struggles, it can help to remember "just like me."

You can say to yourself:

> My child, just like all children, will have struggles, and just like me, all parents worry about their children.
> Just like me, all parents find parenting really difficult at times.
> Just like me, all parents sometimes feel they could have handled something better than they did.
> Just like me, all parents want their children to be happy.
> Just like me, all parents feel bad when their child is hurt (disappointed, sad, lonely . . .)
> Just like me (*add your own words here*).

In those cases when self-judgment is strong, we could also say to ourselves, with so much kindness and understanding:

> How human of me.

I find this phrase, used by author and yoga teacher Judith Lasater, so helpful, and I am grateful to the person who shared it in the chat during an online training I attended.

WE CAN ALWAYS BEGIN AGAIN

In addition to the "just like me" messages, you could also remind yourself that you can always begin again. Sharon Salzberg, the meditation teacher and expert on loving-kindness practice, often uses this phrase in her meditations. In discussing her book *Real Life: The Journey from Isola-*

tion to Openness and Freedom, she highlighted the importance of this skill, saying, "It is the coming back that matters. Beginning again is a training in resilience. We fall, we get up, and we start again." In life, as in formal meditation practice, we can begin again; each moment is a new beginning. If it is appropriate for the circumstances, apologize and make amends. Admit if you lost your temper, made an unwise decision, or responded in an unhelpful way. Try to be really gentle with yourself. Then, with kindness, begin again. If you are caught in a story, you can say to yourself, "It's okay, honey. Begin again." Or use a more forceful approach as you tell yourself kindly and firmly to drop the story and begin again.

Our Reactivity to Others' Struggles

Being truly present with anyone in a moment of distress can be incredibly difficult and uncomfortable. This discomfort often leads us to habitual reactive ways of relating to that individual. We may struggle to search for the "right thing" to say, feel flooded by our emotions, or even numb out to avoid the intensity. We all have our habitual ways of handling these situations. When our child struggles, for all the reasons mentioned and more, our reactivity can be harder to work with, as the intensity of our emotions is often amplified.

It can be helpful to look for reactive tendencies in less intense situations to begin to see them more clearly. At a meeting I attended, a colleague shared, with some visible emotion, her distress and frustration about some ongoing struggles in our community. Almost immediately someone chimed in and minimized the situation to try to make her feel better—a well-intentioned and unnecessary effort to rescue her from her feelings. It can be useful to be on the lookout for times when we do this, both in general and especially with our children. This is a habit that I continue to work with in my life. Though it is a very human response, it can inhibit creating a space where difficult emotions can be seen, named, and felt. Be kind and gentle with yourself if you notice this habit, remembering that it is a totally understandable reaction to intense emotions. As we see this and other habits more clearly and kindly with mindfulness, they start to loosen their hold and can eventually fall away.

SETTLE BACK AND SOFTEN

Leaning, or settling, back is an instruction my teacher gave me several years ago that has been tremendously helpful in working with reactivity when someone else is having a hard time. When someone we care about is struggling, it is not uncommon to experience a feeling of contraction in our body and a physical and energetic sense of leaning forward. You might check in with yourself to see if this is true for you, especially if it is your child who is having a tough time.

In this practice, we consciously reverse that embodied reactivity to our child's difficulties by physically and energetically settling back and inviting the body to soften. The practices of settling back and softening can be beneficial when used separately or in combination. It can be helpful to practice when not in the midst of a challenging situation to begin developing the capacity to remember to settle back and soften when a difficult moment arises.

Try the practice below to begin cultivating a more spacious and receptive state in the body, mind, and heart.

Close your eyes if you are comfortable doing so, taking a few gentle breaths. Think of a time when you felt some reactivity. Pick something on the milder side to begin working with this practice. As you bring the situation to mind, pay attention to how your body feels when recalling this experience. Now, gently and intentionally lean back just a bit. Does anything shift inside of you with this change of your posture? Check in with your body, heart, and mind to see how settling back feels for you.

Next, invite your body to soften and release any unnecessary holding or tension. Soften your jaw and face, your shoulders and chest area, your belly, your back, and your legs. Imagine your whole body is releasing like ice melting into water. Scan your body, heart, and mind to notice how you feel now. Remember, however you feel, that's okay.

The pause between reactive and responsive is the beginning of choice, intention, and skillfulness as a parent.

—*Daniel J. Siegel and Tina Payne Bryson*

Snowplow and Helicopter Parenting

I will never forget hearing the term *snowplow parenting* for the first time. It immediately resonated with me. Yes, I was—and sometimes still am—that parent who tries to get in front of and push away any possible problem for my children. This is snowplow parenting, making the road ahead as smooth and clear as possible. Like *helicopter parenting*, another term commonly used, it is a strategy based on our concern that our child can't manage the difficult situation or the ensuing feelings. Our fear and worry take over, and we opt to micromanage the situation with the best intentions for our child's well-being.

Of course, we need to use wise discernment as well. Knowing those moments when intervening is essential to support our child when they do not have the inner resources to meet a situation. Yet many of us do this without realizing or understanding its problematic nature. By clearing the way or hovering to swoop in and solve problems, we give our children the unhelpful message that we do not trust their capacity to handle their difficulties and emotions. Unfortunately, they may internalize that message and learn not to trust their own inner ability as we deny them the opportunity to flex the muscle of being with difficulties, which enhances their resiliency.

Minimizing, Fixing, Advice-Giving, and Denying

Like so many parents, you may have said to your child, "That's nothing to worry about," or "I am sure they didn't mean to hurt your feelings." These are among a long list of common responses to moments of difficulty that can inadvertently minimize or invalidate our children's experiences and feelings.

Maybe you told your child they are better at something than they are in an effort to bolster their esteem when they compare themselves to others. Or possibly, like so many of us, you may have responded to your child's difficulties by trying to fix a situation or by giving advice. To work with that particular habit, it can help to think of how you feel when someone gives you unsolicited advice and also notice how your child responds when you do it with them. Again, some discernment is needed as there are times when, as an adult, sprinkling a little wisdom and experience is beneficial. Those times are probably less often, however, than you think.

Though understandable and typically well-intentioned, these strategies for trying to manage our children's difficulties come with consequences. When chronic, these ways of relating to our children can leave them feeling unseen and misunderstood without growing their capacity for managing their emotions.

As you practice being on the lookout for some of these habitual ways of reacting to your children's emotions, go gently and do so kindly. (If needed, refer back to working with judgment and shame.) It helps to know that, until we see it clearly, much of our parenting style is out of our control and is influenced by our physiology, our upbringing, and our personal experiences. You are simply paying closer attention and offering kindness to yourself with whatever you notice as you slowly work to change some of the habits that may not be serving you or your child as well as you would like.

Weathering the Storms and Deepening the Roots of Well-Being

Regardless of what they are, our coping skills can have an unintended impact on our children. We want our children to be firmly rooted and to continuously enhance their capacity for handling big and difficult feelings. We want to help them understand that all their feelings belong, are informative, come and go, and are workable.

Our ability to stand our ground and hold space for them in the midst of emotional upheaval is essential to their well-being and ours. As Jon Kabat-Zinn says, "You can't stop the waves, but you can learn how to surf." Our job is to teach our children to see the waves clearly, to give them surfing lessons, and, of course, to be there lovingly when they get knocked over by a wave or two.

PARENTING FROM LOVE

In our concern for our children, we sometimes respond from a place of fear and worry as we lose touch with the love that lies beneath it. Connecting with that love and the wish for our children to be happy and well, especially in moments of difficulty, can be incredibly beneficial. The following practice can support parenting from love.

Begin with a brief mindfulness practice, closing your eyes if that works for you. Once you have settled in and taken a few gentle breaths, shift your attention to think about your child, maybe even picturing them in your imagination. You could call up a time when you experienced warm and loving feelings toward them, noticing what they were doing and remembering how you felt at that time. Now imagine someone has asked you what you love about your child. What words, phrases, images, or descriptions come to mind? Gently check in to notice how you feel in your body, mind, and heart, and rest here for at least three to five breaths to take it in.

This practice is a powerful way to reconnect with feelings of love and cut through the worry and fears that we often experience as parents. It can be helpful to do this as a brief daily practice for a while so you can more easily call up those feelings of love and connection, even in the midst of a challenging moment, before moving on to the next part of the practice.

Once you feel you can readily connect with this love, think of a time when your child was struggling—maybe that's happening now. You can also do this as an informal practice in the midst of some struggle. Then call up the love, reminding yourself of all the things you love about your child. You might even offer them some wishes of well-being and happiness. If the situation calls for you to respond in some way, ask yourself, "How would love respond?" before responding to your child in this situation.

I started using this practice when my daughter was in middle school. When I remembered to use it, I found it incredibly powerful. Although my response to her often didn't change, how I said it, how I felt inside, and how it was received changed quite dramatically and in such a helpful way. Of course, as I mentioned, I didn't always remember, and that's okay. This is simply another reminder that it is all a practice. Sometimes we remember, and sometimes we don't. Be gentle with yourself and keep in mind that falling into old habits is okay, to be expected, and simply a part of parenting and being human.

ONE FOR ME AND ONE FOR YOU

The giving-and-receiving compassion practice is one of my favorite practices from the Mindful Self-Compassion program and one I frequently use when a loved one, friend, or colleague is struggling. I often feel others' pain deeply, which can be draining, difficult, and also not helpful to them. This is especially true when the person struggling is one of my children. In those cases, this practice has made all the difference. You can sit and do this intentionally as a formal practice; as you become more accustomed to the practice, you can do it informally in the midst of a difficult moment.

Begin this practice by closing your eyes if you like. Bring your attention to the sensations of your breath moving in and out of the body, staying with the gentle flow for several breaths. Now think of something your child is struggling with at this time, then consider what it is that *you* most need to support them. It could be strength, balance, calm, acceptance . . . Envision that you are taking that in for yourself as you inhale, then gently release the breath as you exhale.

After doing that for some time, consider what *they* most need amid this difficulty. It could be something different or the same thing you need. Continue to give yourself what you need on the inhale and offer them what they need on the exhale—one for me and one for you. Sometimes I even drop the specific words; as I breathe in and out, I say to myself, "One for me . . . and one for you."

Attitudes and Practices to Support Our Intention

Certain attitudes can deepen our capacity to be in alignment with our intention: being interested and curious about our experience, being receptive and open to trying new things, and always deferring to being gentle and kind with ourselves as we develop new habits of relating to difficulties. We are all learning.

Maybe in our garden we need to have a little reinforcement as we plant the seeds and support the growth of this self-compassionate way of being with ourselves and our children—some stakes in the ground to hold up this intention. The following practices can be helpful to support us in this way.

CALLING IN YOUR WISEST SELF

This practice is adapted from a guided visualization that I experienced at a workshop with the meditation teacher and author Jack Kornfield and one that is included in his book *A Lamp in the Darkness: Illuminating the Path through Difficult Times.*

Close your eyes if you like, and take a few gentle breaths. Bring to mind a deeply wise and caring person. It could be a spiritual figure, a person from your life, a teacher, or even an imaginary being. Picture them as clearly as you can, even imagining how they look at you and how it feels to be in their presence.

Now call to mind a time when you were having a challenging moment with your child. It can help to begin with a mildly difficult moment to support getting accustomed to this practice. Freeze the experience and imagine that wise being offering to become you and help with this situation. Notice what they say and do, paying particular attention to how it feels in your body as you experience the situation from their perspective. Let the felt sense of being "the wise one" soak in. How does your body feel? How about your heart and mind? Remember that this being is always available within you; this is your wisest self. With practice, you will increasingly remember and be able to call on your wisest self in moments of difficulty.

CREATING YOUR VILLAGE

I have always loved the concept of creating a village and have intentionally tried to cultivate a village of wise adults to support my family. The ideal village includes people who are supportive in a variety of ways: some who are the wisdom keepers; some who remind us to see the joy in life; and some who are the coaches, mentors, cheerleaders, caretakers, and helpers. There are those who provide skills and encouragement and those who are deep listeners. Take a moment to think of the individuals and the types of people you want to surround yourself with on this journey of parenting.

You can also gather this village internally. If you like, close your eyes and visualize creating your village. Who do you want to include? The inhabitants can include real people and those from your imagination. Picture them as best as you can and notice what they say or do when you are experiencing a difficult moment with your child. Now check in and see how you feel in your body, mind, and heart when they are supporting you. You might even take time to journal as you reflect on creating your village. Think specifically about when it may be most helpful for them to show up for you.

BE KIND TO YOURSELF

Most importantly, remember that if your child is having a hard time, you are also suffering and need to care for yourself. This can include practicing the skills highlighted in chapter 2 as you offer yourself kindness and care—a touch of mindfulness and self-compassion can go far. When things are hard for your child, being kind to yourself is always a good place to start.

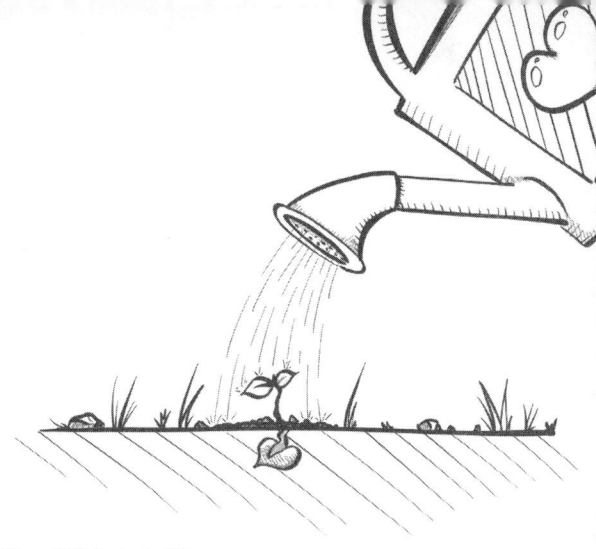

PART TWO

Watering the Flowers: Nurturing Self-Compassion in Children

4

Why Children Need
Self-Compassion

HELPING CHILDREN MANAGE difficult experiences and emotions is more crucial than ever. Children's mental health issues were on the rise from 2016 to 2020, according to a study showing a significant increase in depression and anxiety.[5] Since that time, we have only begun to assess the impact of COVID-19 on children's mental health. A survey of thirty-five studies regarding child and adolescent mental health during the pandemic showed COVID-19's concerning impact on well-being, indicating that anxiety, depression, loneliness, stress, and tension are the most observed symptoms.[6]

This research is certainly reflected in my (Wendy's) experience working with children, parents, educators, and nonprofit professionals. I see an increasing number of children who are struggling to manage their feelings, overwhelmed, and often anxious. Many lack effective socialization and coping skills. For those children with a diminished capacity to handle life's difficulties, circumstances that may have caused minimal stress in the past have become experiences of deep distress.

Why do we need to pay attention to these facts, which can, honestly, be so hard to hear? First, it is helpful to know that if your child is struggling, you are not alone. This powerful reminder of our common humanity can decrease isolation during difficult times. With a basic understanding of what is happening for children in general and taking the time to consider how it impacts our children specifically, we can also begin to see ways to address these concerns.

Supporting our children requires a willingness to see their difficulties clearly and to find the middle path of not being overwhelmed by the challenges before us but also not being in denial of the support that is needed at this time for our children. As we look at some of what is happening more broadly in our society, you may reflect on how your child manages the ups and downs in these areas of life and what might be helpful. In my experience, self-compassion is a powerful path forward and a beautiful gift we can give our children.

The professional development session I was scheduled to facilitate for early childhood educators at the start of the COVID-19 pandemic was canceled and eventually moved online. As I prepared, I reflected on what was needed and how my time with these adults could best benefit them and the children in their care. In particular, I considered what I was finding most helpful for my own well-being. Like so many others, the shutdown during the pandemic and all its ramifications deeply affected me. As I acknowledged how I was struggling, I began, with more intention, to bring much-needed kindness and loving awareness to myself and my experience. With self-compassion becoming my new default, I often found myself saying with a hand on my heart, "Of course you are feeling this way, honey. It's okay. I am right here." At this moment my book *It's OK: Being Kind to Yourself When Things Feel Hard* was born. I realized, for many reasons, that though this moment certainly called for mindfulness, heavy doses of self-compassion were the priority for adults and children.

This section of the book will dive into the question "How can I support my child in being with their difficulties?" Understanding some of the specific struggles enhances our awareness of the vital role that self-compassion can play and ways to share it most effectively with our children.

There are, of course, many reasons why children are struggling at this time. I will highlight just a few that can explicitly benefit from being held with the kindness and care of a self-compassionate perspective and share some ways to address them in our efforts to support children's happiness and resilience. Here we include a few practices to begin exploring these topics, with many more to come in the following chapters.

The Winds of Disconnection

The pandemic intensified what has been called a loneliness epidemic in our society, with many of us feeling more disconnected than ever. In addition, societal pressure for external achievement and moving quickly toward the next goal or scheduled activity leaves little time to "just be" and "to be with" one another. We are bombarded with messages encouraging us to acquire things in order to be happy and well. This focus on collecting instead of connecting doesn't support prioritizing the development of meaningful relationships but instead encourages our sense of self and happiness to depend on what we have, look like, and achieve.

Social media, a mainstay in our children's lives, reinforces this focus on appearances—often not accurate ones—instead of deep and meaningful connections. In his statement about the increase in loneliness in America, US Surgeon General Vivek Murthy warned that many young people now use social media as a replacement for in-person relationships. This often leads to lower-quality connections.[7] We are inherently social creatures, and children need loving and authentic connections to thrive.

Our efforts to reverse this trend of loneliness, isolation, and our diminishing sense of connection can greatly benefit from a self-compassion practice, as well as help us in developing one. When we recognize and actively cultivate a sense of our shared humanity, an aspect of self-compassion, our loneliness decreases and our capacity for self-compassion increases. They are mutually supportive tools. The practice of self-compassion can be a beautiful reminder that we are all connected, make mistakes, struggle at times, and are worthy of kindness and care.

THE CONNECTION REFLECTION

In his book *Hardwiring Happiness: The New Brain Science of Contentment, Calm, and Confidence*, the author and neuroscientist Rick Hanson identifies three basic human needs: safety, satisfaction, and connection. In his Foundations of Well-Being course, he highlights feeling included, seen, liked, appreciated, loved, compassionate, kind, and generous as key resources to support the need for connection.

You might take some time to reflect or journal about how you can support your child in these areas. Look for ways to help them feel seen, liked, appreciated, and loved. This could be in the way that you respond to them or drawing their attention to it in relation to how they are connecting with others. For example, you might say, "I noticed how Auntie Debbie loves to spend time with you and how much she appreciates your imaginative stories and silly times together." Similarly, be sure not to miss it when they act in compassionate, kind, and generous ways, even naming those moments for them. For example, if they share a toy with a sibling, you might say to them, "How kind of you to share your toy with your sister."

The way we relate to our children supports their inner voice. If we can help them to see and feel connection in their lives, they can internalize this powerful capacity for well-being.

OFFERING KINDNESS TO OTHERS

Having children wish others well is another way to support this internal sense of connection and deepen their understanding of common humanity. The meditation teacher Sharon Salzberg is well known for these teachings, and her book *Loving-Kindness: The Revolutionary Art of Happiness* is a great resource if you want to dive deeper. Here are a few ideas to begin.

You can use a bowl and some stones to develop a ritual of well-wishing. Ask your child to think about someone they are close to as they hold a stone. They could even close their eyes to see if they can picture this person. While holding the stone, they can make a wish such as "May you be happy and well" and then put the stone in the bowl. Other variations could be "May you be safe and healthy," "May your heart be filled with love," "May you be peaceful," or any wish they want to use. If the phrase "May you . . ." feels awkward, they could simply use the phrase "I wish you . . ."—for example, "I wish you happiness."

Invite your child to do this for a few special people, then move on to a few people that they do not know well and repeat the process. Next, include one or two people that they may sometimes find difficult. Finally, have them put in a stone, sending wishes to everyone everywhere.

This is a lovely practice to do with them or even to do together as a family. You and your child can also draw hearts on the stones or decorate them in some way that reminds you of wishing others well. Be sure to pause and have them notice how it feels for them emotionally and in their body when they offer kindness to others.

Another option is to do this with your child throughout the day. You can support your child in silently sending kind wishes to people they see while going about their day, such as people walking down the street, in cars nearby, in school, or in stores. Again, encourage your child to notice how their body feels and even the impact on their emotions when they offer kindness to others. As they see someone, encourage them to say to themselves, "May you be happy" or "I wish you happiness," recognizing that all people want and deserve to be happy and well. I sometimes do this practice as I pass homes when I drive, offering the wish "May you be joyful" to all the people inside. When I am having a bout of grouchy feelings, this practice for connection and common humanity is at the top of my list.

The Winds of Unworthiness or Not Good Enough

In my work with families, I often hear young people say they feel "less than" or just "not good enough" as they unfavorably compare themselves to others. This sense of unworthiness is so painful for children and is heightened by the cultural focus on achievement and competition, high-lighting external instead of intrinsic value. Like us, our children experi-ence social pressure to strive to be or get more, to be or do better, and generally to be other than they are.

These feelings of "not good enough" can be subtle, and yet they can have a powerful impact. It is helpful to see how this affects our children, including how we relate to them. As we try to help our children grow and develop, we can look out for any messages that they are not enough or need to be fixed. With caring acceptance, we can help them to hold their mistakes and struggles kindly, encouraging growth from that place of love and care.

As the esteemed psychologist Carl Rogers said, "The curious paradox is that when I can accept myself, just as I am, then I can change."[8] This perspective—accepting and welcoming it all, including all the messiness in our lives, with as much tenderness and care as possible—is integrated into mindfulness and self-compassion teaching. To teach this to our children, we must model and remind them of it. Though stated before, I believe we as caregivers can't be reminded enough that this also holds true for us. There is messiness, mistake-making, comparing, and feelings of not being good enough in parenting. What a gift it would be to our children if we could use those moments to truly and authentically model self-compassion as we remember that we are parenting, not perfecting.

> Imperfection is not our personal problem—it is a natural part of existing.
>
> —*Tara Brach*

The Winds of Adversity

All families and all children deal with adversity in varying degrees. Dif-ficult situations impact both adults and children. Often, amid stress, the fight-flight-freeze response activates in an effort to keep us safe. In some situations, this activation can help us deal with the difficulty at hand. Yet for far too many of us, it can get stuck there, shifting us into this place of heightened arousal, anxiety, and activation for too long and too easily.

We also have another way of responding to stress: the affiliate stress response, or tend and befriend. This stress response focuses on social support and connection. As parents, we can help our children tap into the affiliate stress response as we support them when they are struggling. Here we offer you some ways to do just that.

What really intrigued me when I first learned the terminology for the affiliate response was the fact that these same words, *tend and befriend*, are also often used in reference to mindfulness and self-compassion practices—*tend* being the mindfulness aspect, and *befriend* the offering of compassion and kindness. Though the affiliate response is typically referred to in terms of external social connection, in my experience, instilling the capacity for self-compassion can greatly support children in this way as they learn to tend and befriend themselves through hard times.

HOLD IT IN A LOVING HEART

For the Hold It in a Loving Heart activity, decorate or make a heart-shaped container. You can use clay or another material, or use a paper plate and decorate it with a heart. On slips of paper, have your child write or create visual expressions of difficult experiences and the related feelings they noticed. (Younger children can stick pictures onto paper.) Then have them place the slips of paper in the container or on the plate to symbolize holding the difficulty with care and kindness in a loving heart. As they put the paper in the container or on the plate, support them in saying, "I can hold this hard feeling in my kind and loving heart"; or they can say, "I care about this difficulty and can hold it kindly in my heart." For younger children, you could support them to say, "This is hard, and I can give this hard thing lots of kindness."

This is also an opportunity to begin conversations about ways to offer themselves kindness in the midst of difficulties. You can ask them if there are ways that they can give themselves kindness when things are hard.

Ideas might be getting a hug, playing with some favorite toys, or snuggling up with a pet. You might suggest they check in with how their body feels when giving themselves and their tricky moment kindness, maybe offering some prompts like, "Does it feel warm?" "Does your body feel soft?" "Do you feel cozy?" Another option is to read the papers in the heart at the end of the day or once a week as a family and offer one another some gestures of compassion (a hug or kind words) to support internalizing messages of loving-kindness.

The Winds of Negativity

In his explanation of the negativity bias, Rick Hanson talks about how we are wired so that negative experiences stick like Velcro and positive experiences slide off like Teflon. Though helpful from an evolutionary standpoint, this bias is not so helpful for our ongoing happiness. Our nervous system is wired to focus on, more easily remember, and even scan for negative experiences or problems. Like us, our children have this bias, and they often get stuck ruminating about unpleasant and difficult experiences, which impacts their happiness, mental health, and well-being. Knowing this, we can give our children tools to actively take in positive experiences and teach them to access their internal caregiving network when negative experiences dominate their attention.

SOAK IT IN: TAKING LOVE AND KINDNESS INTO OUR HEARTS

In his book *Awakening through Love: Unveiling Your Deepest Goodness*, the meditation teacher and theology professor John Makransky states that "many of us haven't learned to pay much attention to the countless moments of love, kindness, and care that surrounds us each day." He encourages us to see the love that is always coming toward us. We want to help our children to be on the lookout for that kindness and to soak it into their bodies, hearts, and minds. This is a powerful way to combat the negativity bias, support a sense of loving connection, and internalize feelings of love and care for ourselves. The following practice is an adaptation of Makransky's practice of receiving love and the practice of "taking in the good" from Rick Hanson's work.

To prepare for this practice, take a sponge and cut it into the shape of a heart and/or write "Soak it in" on the sponge with a permanent marker. You can do this with your child as you talk about how our brains are so busy trying to help us avoid problems that sometimes we miss the good stuff. We are going to practice being on the lookout for the good and soaking it in, and our heart sponge will be a helpful reminder.

At the beginning of the day, talk to your child about being a "kindness detector," which means being on the lookout for kindness throughout the day. This doesn't have to be a big gesture of kindness; it could be a smile, someone saying hello, holding a door, someone showing interest in what you are doing, someone sharing at school, or any other offering of goodwill or kindness. This expression of care could come from a family member, a friend, an acquaintance, or even a stranger. It may be acts of warmth or appreciation directed at them or that they witness between others. This is an opportunity to help them appreciate that we are all surrounded by love and care. It is part of the air we all breathe. When you are with your child, you can support them in noticing by pointing out these examples as they happen.

I suggest doing this practice toward the end of the day. It can be done with your child individually by having them share step 1 aloud and then leading them through the other steps for them to do silently. Alternatively, you could do this as a family activity by making a sponge for each family member. Do the first step aloud by going around and sharing and then cueing the other four steps, which everyone could do simultaneously and silently.

Tell them that each time they squeeze the sponge it is a reminder that, like a sponge, they can soak feelings of love and care into their hearts, filling up their hearts with kindness. Ask them to hold their sponge and recall one experience of love or kindness that they noticed that day and do the following practice.

1. Share the experience and then squeeze the sponge as a reminder to let the good feelings soak into your heart—filling yourself with feelings of kindness and care.
2. Remember as much detail as possible, using all your senses, then squeeze the sponge again.
3. Notice how it feels in your body when someone is kind, then squeeze the sponge for the third time.
4. Imagine letting that feeling fill your body. Then squeeze the sponge again to encourage soaking it in more deeply.
5. Tell your brain this feeling is worth keeping as you squeeze the sponge for a final time.

What about Self-Esteem?

Parents and teachers often ask me about self-esteem. Self-esteem is, by virtue of its nature, often dependent on external conditions. For example, our child's self-esteem can be boosted by a good grade, an achievement in sports or some other activity, or some positive feedback. Trying to bolster our child's self-esteem, we might tell them they are good at something, typically connected to an achievement and often based on comparison with others. Self-esteem is available when things are going well and not usually accessible to us in the midst of a difficult moment when we need it most.

Self-compassion, however, is based on our intrinsic value as human beings. Like all humans, we struggle, mess up, and have a hard time occasionally, and we all deserve kindness simply because we are struggling. There is nothing else required for us to access this beneficial tool. Imagine the possible far-reaching benefits of developing a skill that is based on common humanity and kindness as opposed to competition and comparison.

I can certainly feel this difference and encourage you to reflect on it as well. When a child struggles, instead of trying to convince them that they are the best at something or better than someone else, we can start by acknowledging how hard it is to feel like they are not good enough. We can help them learn to bring kindness and care to the difficult moment and their feelings instead of trying to make it go away with often futile efforts to boost their self-esteem.

For example, suppose your child says that their friend is better at soccer, which may in fact be true. Instead of pretending it isn't true and trying to build them up, you could start by acknowledging their feelings. For instance, you might say, "It sounds like you are feeling bad about how you are doing at soccer. It's really hard to feel that way." Alternatively, you could say, "It's really hard to feel like you aren't as good as someone else." As we dive into the other aspects of self-compassion, we will share how to extend this discussion and, as appropriate, remind our children of common humanity and ways to practice offering themselves some kindness.

Self-Compassion to Tend to the Flowers

Considering the influences on our children's well-being mentioned above, effectively introducing self-compassion practices to children and integrating these practices into family life can be tremendously beneficial. As was mentioned before, research has shown that the ability to be self-compassionate is linked to greater emotional resilience and psychological well-being in a variety of ways. Specific research with adolescents has found that self-compassion is a skill that can be learned and that it is correlated with increased life satisfaction and decreased anxiety and depression.[9]

Additionally, research on post-traumatic stress disorder (PTSD) shows that self-compassion can be a helpful intervention and a protective factor, meaning those with higher levels of self-compassion were shown to be less likely to develop PTSD symptoms following a traumatic experience.[10] Self-compassion also supports developing a growth mindset.[11] In her book *Mindset: The New Psychology of Success*, the psychologist Carol Dweck highlights the benefits of a growth mindset, a belief that abilities and personality traits are malleable and that there is always potential to grow and improve.

Because there is limited research on self-compassion with children, the research highlighted here is specific to adults and adolescents. However, based on our many years of working with children, we strongly believe they also experience these benefits. We look forward to more research to support our anecdotal experience. In my life, the power of bringing love and care to suffering cannot be overstated. With self-compassion in my back pocket, I ride the ups and downs of life with much more ease. With self-compassion now in my parenting toolbox, I hope to continue to help my children, now adults, to do the same.

As my colleague Zahabiyah Yamasaki, a trauma-informed yoga educator and author, said to me, "Children are born beautiful and whole, but the world presents systemic conditions that can challenge their capacity for coping. Yes, children are resilient, and they are worthy of tender, compassionate, and trauma-informed support to remind them how loved, enough, and not alone they are." We can offer that support to them and, as we teach them self-compassion, help them learn how to offer it to themselves.

Sharing Self-Compassion with Children: Sprinkling and Watering the Seeds

When I teach about mindfulness and self-compassion, I often use the analogy of sprinkling seeds as we consider how to create the best conditions for self-compassion to grow. Though many parents are eager to support their children and share these practices, I encourage them to go gently and slowly, keeping this idea of sprinkling seeds in mind. If we are overzealous, though well-intentioned, we can easily crush the seeds. Keep it light, even fun and playful, and please do not make self-compassion another thing to accomplish. Learning happens through play and during times of connection. We want to develop our children's curiosity and interest in their inner experience, not make it something they feel pressured to do. On the other hand, if we do not plant the seeds, nothing grows, so some intention, as was previously mentioned, is needed.

The sprinkling takes place as we practice. This can be formal practices as well as the integration of self-compassion into daily life, including ways of talking to children that support them in developing this deep sense of self-kindness.

Capture teachable moments as they happen, and sprinkle practices throughout the day, little bits often, to help self-compassion become a way of life for you and your family. Weave it in as you read a book, play a game, watch a show, or talk about the stories of the day. Your modeling matters, so do not hesitate to show ways that you are practicing as well. With mindfulness and self-compassion, we gently share practices and then let go, being cautious not to focus on results. Meeting children where they are is essential and something I stress in my teaching. It is important not to correct, critique, or push in any way. If you sense resistance, be sensitive to their timing and pace and follow their lead. Remember that children, like all of us, have very complex inner worlds, and we want to respect their inner experiences and life situations.

When teaching a first-grade class, I invited everyone to sit up tall before moving into a breathing practice. One little boy was, once again, mostly slouched down in his chair. The teacher started to head over to correct him, and I caught her eye and let her know he was just fine as he was. Weeks later, I was told that this little one's mom had called the school to express gratitude for the mindfulness skills her son was now using to help him as they dealt with a difficult family situation. Allowing children to access the practices when and how they can is one way we show them kindness and compassion. Remember, even with our own children, we never know what is going on inside another person, and we need to tread gently.

It is important that we do not wait for them to be in crisis to begin practicing self-compassion. The analogy of the piano is once again helpful. We wouldn't practice a song on the piano for the first time at the concert. We would practice it many times, so it becomes second nature. Similarly, we practice self-compassion in various ways and initially use it with minor difficulties so that it becomes second nature and is easier to do when a truly difficult moment arises. As we practice, we are developing the pathways in our brain that support our ability and our children's ability to respond in this way with presence, connection, and self-kindness.

WHAT WE PRACTICE GROWS

This activity helps children understand that what we practice is what we grow in our lives. On a paper cup, write the words "What we practice grows stronger." Explain that if we want to get better at something, it is important that we practice. You can use examples from various aspects of life, such as playing a sport or an instrument or engaging in creative activities like art. Invite your child to remember a time that they practiced really hard at something and to remember how the practice helped them.

Then explain that the same is true for what we want to grow inside of us—things like kindness, patience, gratitude, love, and joy. To grow them, it helps to pay attention and do things that help us practice them. For example, if we want to grow gratitude, we may practice by writing down things we are grateful for or, at the end of the day, sharing something we are grateful for as a family.

You can do this project focusing on any of the inner qualities that you want to cultivate, like those mentioned above. For our purposes, we will do this activity focusing on growing self-compassion. Have your child cut out the shape of a flower using some sturdy paper. In the center of the flower, write "self-compassion" or "self-kindness" and glue it onto a popsicle stick for a stem. They can plant the flower in the cup using sand to hold it in.

Next, have them decorate stones and write on them some of the ways that they will grow self-compassion. What might they practice that will help them? Some examples include the three parts of self-compassion: noticing when things are hard, remembering everyone has a hard time sometimes, and treating yourself like a good friend. Or it could be specific ways they will be kind to themselves, such as talking to themselves kindly, placing a hand on their heart, getting a hug (or hugging a stuffed animal or pet), or snuggling up in a blanket. Spend some time together coming up with ways they can practice being kind to themselves. For younger children, you can also decorate the stones with images instead of words to remind them of how they will practice being kind to themselves. Possibly a picture of a heart or a pet or even some letters to represent talking kindly to themselves. It can also help to share, as appropriate, some ways that you are practicing being kind to yourself. Consider making your own "self-compassion" flower and stones and do this project together.

Put the stones around the "flowerpot" to serve as a visual cue, helping keep the attention and intention focused on growing self-compassion. They could even add small stones to the cup each time they do something to practice and grow this skill with the reminder that they are strengthening it each time they drop another stone in to support the flower.

5

Mindfulness:
The Light of Awareness

IN CHAPTER 2 we introduced how to nurture our own mindfulness practice. Here we will explore how to introduce mindfulness-based practices to children. Mindfulness is the cultivation of present-moment awareness—what is happening in our internal world and externally around us. As we shine that light of awareness on our inner world, we begin to cultivate an attunement and intimacy with ourselves; we begin to deeply know ourselves.

One way that I (Louise) like to describe mindfulness is by imagining a window of awareness in our mind through which we perceive the world. Research tells us that our attention wanders away from the present moment about 47 percent of the time, so we can imagine that almost half of that window is fogged up.[12] As we practice mindfulness, it is a bit like clearing off the fog from that window, bit by bit, so that more and more of our lives and ourselves become available to us.

Self-compassion means bringing kindness to ourselves during moments of suffering. In order to give ourselves this kindness, we need to know that we are, in fact, suffering. As we cultivate more presence in our inner and outer lives, we are able to notice these moments of difficulty as they happen and then meet ourselves with kindness, gentleness, and care. Mindfulness also helps us relate to challenging moments and difficult emotions with nonjudgment and acceptance. Rather than resisting discomfort, we can allow it to simply be there, letting go of trying to battle with it or push it away. As we do this, we can meet difficult moments with much more ease and spaciousness. So, in this way, the cultivation of mindful presence is the foundation for our self-compassion practice.

I can honestly say that learning how to meditate has been one of the most transformational experiences of my life so far. Although I had spent years studying psychology, it was only when I started to meditate that I began to truly know myself and to understand the nature of my mind. It was such a huge relief to learn that although we can't always control the circumstances of our lives, we always have a choice in how we respond to those circumstances. This is the gift that mindfulness practice brings us. Developing this understanding that we have a choice in how we respond to our inner and outer experiences was then, and continues to be, deeply empowering for me.

After experiencing the profound benefits of mindfulness in my early twenties, I began to wonder how my life would have been different if I had been introduced to this practice in my earlier years. Although I had achieved very well academically throughout my life, from around the age of eight I experienced persistent anxiety and periods of unhappiness. As I journeyed deeper with my meditation practice, receiving so many benefits along the way, I became frustrated that many school systems are so heavily focused on academic and sporting achievement. I never remember once being asked at school how I was feeling. My experience throughout my education was as if my internal world had little importance. Of course, we need to support children's academic learning, but I passionately feel that supporting children's positive mental health and well-being is also of utmost importance. After all, isn't happiness what we all most deeply want for our children?

Spurred by this deep wish to support children's emotional well-being, I began sharing mindfulness-based practices with children. I developed Creative Mindfulness Kids, a method for sharing mindfulness and compassion-based practices with children in creative, playful, and child-friendly ways. It has been such a deep honor to have trained so many others around the world in facilitating this work with children.

Creative Activities and Practices

The term *mindfulness* is quite an abstract concept. It can be difficult for even some adults to understand. However, by learning mindfulness through the use of colorful props and creative activities, children can experience the practice in a very tangible way. Their understanding of mindfulness-based concepts is thus developed and nurtured experientially. When children take the time to make their own mindfulness crafts, it becomes something very personal and meaningful for them.

The crafts can also be taken out and interacted with frequently, so they promote the cultivation of a regular mindfulness practice. I have lost count of the number of times parents have told me that their child still treasures their "Creative Mindfulness" crafts years after we had made them together. The creative activities also support parental involvement in their child's mindfulness practices. Children and parents can explore the crafts together, and parents can even make their own crafts alongside their children.

Though previous chapters have included some creative-based activities to support the development of self-compassion for children, the remainder of the book will have even more opportunities to teach children about self-compassion in this way. With that in mind, it is helpful to have an understanding of how to best use these creative practice offerings.

What is always most important is that we ourselves do our best to embody a loving, connected presence as we guide children through the activities. We can also use this time as a chance to practice mindfulness informally, noticing when we become distracted and then bringing our focus gently back to our child and the activity. Remember that every new moment is an opportunity to begin again.

It is important that we always present these activities and practices to children as invitational. Before beginning, check in with your child and ask them whether they would like to try the activity or practice. If they are feeling resistant, it is best to wait and try again another time.

Some of the activities include opportunities for you and your child to reflect and share your experiences, thoughts, and feelings. Check in with your child and ask them whether they would like to share or if they are okay with you sharing. If they seem hesitant, you can come back to this part of the practice another time. During these reflective pieces, it will greatly benefit your child if you do your best to practice listening to them mindfully, with nonjudgment and kindness, giving them lots of time and space to share.

Making your own version of each of the creative activities is a lovely way to support your child while also sharing authentically how the activities support your own cultivation of mindfulness and self-compassion. It is also helpful to encourage your child to notice how they feel in their body, mind, and heart as they engage with the activities and practices. Always assure them that however they feel in any particular moment is okay. You can say to them, "All your feelings are welcome." Your child will benefit from hearing this again and again.

The craft-based activities can be kept together in your child's "special space," which can be a spot that is special to your child somewhere in their home. You and your child can have fun creating and decorating their special space. Some children love creating their own makeshift tent for their special space, using material, blankets, and soft cushions. The most important thing is that the space feels inviting, comfortable, and special for them.

The activities work best when they are practiced frequently, ideally making the activities and practices a regular part of your child's everyday life. As mentioned in chapter 4, we can sprinkle each day with a variety of mindfulness and self-compassion practices, and creative activities can be part of this. The craft pieces and props can be taken out and interacted with regularly, particularly when your child is experiencing difficult emotions or struggling in some way.

MONKEY MIND

As we practice mindfulness, we gain an understanding that our mind tends to wander from the present moment to past and future thoughts. Mindfulness practices deepen our self-awareness around our thoughts. We become familiar with our thinking process and the type of thoughts we think. This activity will support your child to gain a deeper awareness of the nature of their mind and their own thinking process. It will also support you in cultivating a deeper understanding of your child's inner world. You will need a toy monkey, paper, and crayons for this activity.

Begin by showing your child the toy monkey and invite them to give the monkey a name if they like. You can share with them that sometimes it is like we have a busy monkey in our minds. Explain that usually, the monkey doesn't like to keep still and that it can sometimes be a very busy monkey. It likes to jump around to lots of different thoughts. You can play with the monkey, showing how it likes to jump from thought to thought, just like a monkey jumps from tree to tree.

Next, say that sometimes the monkey likes to jump to thoughts about what is going to happen in the future. Give your child some examples of different kinds of future thoughts—for example: What is going to happen next? What am I going to do later? Or thinking about upcoming birthdays or special events. Explain that at other times, the monkey likes to jump to things that have happened in the past. Give your child some examples of different types of past thoughts, such as thinking about what happened yesterday or last week. You can also say that sometimes the monkey jumps to other thoughts, like the things and people we love and are interested in.

The following step is to take some time to share with your child (age appropriately) about where your own monkey mind likes to jump to. You can play with the monkey again to demonstrate this. Now, give the monkey to your child and invite them to share what kind of thoughts their monkey mind jumps to. Give them time and space to share, always listening to them with mindfulness and kindness as best as you can.

You can extend this activity by inviting your child to draw their monkey mind on a blank sheet of paper. Then you can ask them to draw, write, or stick on pictures of the different types of thoughts they think about as their monkey mind jumps around. When they have finished drawing the picture, you can ask them whether they would like to chat with you about what they have drawn or written on their page. This activity works particularly well when it is repeated regularly with your child.

GIVING OUR MONKEY MIND A JOB

Mindfulness practice helps us recognize when we are "thinking," to let go of those thoughts, and to gently return to the present moment. This activity will help your child to understand what the "present moment" means. It will help them use the anchor of their breath to bring their mind to the here and now and to begin a basic mindful breathing practice.

Start by asking your child whether they know what the here and now is. You can explain that the here and now is what is happening in this moment right now. Share that we are in the here and now when we are noticing what we can see, hear, touch, smell, and taste in this moment. Take some time to share with your child what you are noticing in the present moment, and then invite them to share what they are noticing in the here and now.

As in the previous practice, show your child the toy monkey and remind them how our mind is like a monkey who jumps from thought to thought. You can, once again, play with the monkey, making it jump around to demonstrate this. Remind them that the monkey likes to jump to thoughts about the past and future, and when we are thinking about past and future thoughts, we are not in the here and now. Share that a way to look after ourselves well and to be a kind friend to ourselves is to bring our mind into the here and now.

Explain that when we give our monkey mind a job to do, we can help bring it into the here and now. One job we can give our monkey mind is to notice our breathing. Next, invite your child to put their hand on their belly and to close their eyes if they like. Encourage them to notice the feeling of their belly moving as they breathe in and out. Guide them to practice like this for about five breaths at first. You can increase the number of breaths as they practice.

After practicing like this a few times, you can ask your child to pay attention to when their monkey mind jumps away from the breath to thinking about a thought. You can share that when we notice that our monkey mind has jumped to a thought, we can jump it right back to its job of noticing the feeling of our breathing. You can support your child to practice this informally by taking a few mindful breaths together anytime throughout the day or more formally using the following meditation script. Particularly good times to practice mindful breathing with them include before school, transitions throughout the day, before and after mealtimes, and before bed.

MONKEY MIND MEDITATION

The following meditation script is a simple practice to support your child in connecting to their breath and the present moment. You can invite them to sit or lie down as they listen to the meditation, whichever they feel most comfortable with.

MONKEY MIND MEDITATION SCRIPT

Have you ever noticed that your mind can be very busy, like a little monkey sometimes? At times it likes to bounce about thinking—thinking about lots of different things. What does your monkey mind like to think about? Sometimes our monkey mind can get very busy. Do you ever have a busy monkey mind?

Now, we are going to give your monkey mind a job to do. The job is to notice the feeling of your breathing, just noticing the feeling of your breath as you breathe in and out.

Are you ready to have a go?

If you like, you can close your eyes and put your hand on your belly. Can you feel your belly moving as you breathe in and out? Notice your belly moving; just notice your breathing in and your breathing out.

(Pause for ten seconds.)

Are you still feeling your belly moving? If your monkey mind has jumped away and is thinking about a thought, jump it back to its job, just feeling your belly moving as you breathe.

Well done!

Feel your belly get bigger as you breathe in and get smaller as you breathe out. Feel your hands move up and down on your belly as you breathe. Breathing in and breathing out.

Check to see if your monkey mind is still doing its job. Check to see if you are still noticing your breath. If your monkey mind has jumped to a thought, just jump it back to feeling your belly moving as you breathe.

Can you practice this on your own now for a little while?

(Pause for twenty seconds)

Can you notice how you feel inside? How does your head feel? How does your body feel? How does your heart feel? Remember, however you feel right now, that's okay. It is always okay to feel like you do.

When you are ready, you can wriggle your fingers and toes and open your eyes.

THE FIVE SENSES PRACTICE

Mindfulness is about much more than simply noticing our breathing. When we connect to our body and our five senses, we are connecting to the here and now. The body and the senses are always anchored in the now.

Take out the monkey again and explain to your child that we can also give our monkey mind other jobs to do to help bring it into the here and now. Explain that we can give our monkey mind the job of noticing what we can see around us, what we can hear around us, what we can touch, what we can smell, and what we can taste. Share that just like when we are noticing our breath, if we catch our monkey mind jumping away to different thoughts, we can remember to jump it back to its job. Experiment with supporting your child to notice what they are experiencing through their five senses and explain that when they are doing this, they are bringing their mind into the here and now, and they are practicing mindfulness.

Throughout the day, you can pause with your child, take a deep breath together, and invite them to connect to a particular sense. You can ask them questions like:

I wonder what sounds you can hear now?
What colors can you see in this room?
What can you touch in this moment?
Is there anything you can smell right now?
Your child can also ask you questions about what you are experiencing through your senses.

FEELING FRIENDS

As we bring mindful awareness to our inner world, we notice that our thoughts and emotions are impermanent in nature; they are always moving and changing. We also learn to let go of judging our emotions as bad or wrong and instead bring a welcoming acceptance to all of our feelings. This practice supports children to recognize and label their emotions. It also helps them understand the transitory nature of emotions and that all emotions are okay to have.

Begin by taking some time to discuss with your child about the different types of feelings that we can have. Follow up by asking them whether they think it's okay to feel sad, worried, nervous, shy, or angry. Invite your child to consider whether they think there are good or bad feelings and give them plenty of time and space to discuss this with you.

Assure them that all our feelings are okay and that although some emotions might be uncomfortable, all our feelings are important and that we all feel sad, worried, nervous, shy, and angry sometimes. Share with them that our feelings are like visitors; they come to visit us for a while, but they don't stay forever. They always leave again soon. At times, our feelings are very big, at times they are small, and other times they are in between. Explain that each day we get visited by different feelings.

Sometimes we get a visit from just one feeling. Other times, a mixture of feelings visits us. Invite your child to give names to their different feeling visitors—for example, Sad Sandrina, Worried Walter, and Nervous Nelly.

Next, you can encourage your child to notice which feeling or feelings are visiting them at that moment. As they share their feelings with you, try your best to listen to your child with mindfulness and kindness. Then, if it feels appropriate, you can also share what feeling or feelings are currently visiting you. When you have both finished sharing, you can support your child to say:

> (*Insert feeling name*) is visiting me today.
> That is okay. All feelings are okay to have.
> They will be here for a while and will be on their way again soon.

HEART HOUSE AND FEELING VISITORS

The Heart House and Feeling Visitors activity expands on the Feeling Friends practice. It supports children in welcoming and accepting their feelings, particularly uncomfortable emotions. It also deepens their understanding of the impermanent nature of emotions. For this activity, you will need an empty shoebox, crayons, and craft materials such as clay, felt, and sturdy paper.

Encourage your child to reflect on their feelings as visitors and the different names they gave them. Next, invite them to make characters for each of their feeling visitors. Your child can make as many feeling visitors as they like, but try to include characters for sadness, happiness, anger, excitement, shyness, fear, embarrassment, and worry. The characters can be made from clay, sturdy paper, stones, wooden pegs, felt, or other materials. To make the heart house, ask your child to decorate the lid of the shoebox like the front of a house. They can also decorate the inside of the box if they like. Support them in writing the words "All feelings welcome" on the front of the box.

You can explain to your child that it is like there is a little house in their heart, and each day, different feelings come to visit their heart house. The feelings will stay for a while but will soon be on their way again. Share with them that sometimes we have just one feeling visitor, and other times we can have a few feelings visiting us together. The most important thing is to remind them that no matter what feeling comes to visit their heart house, it is always okay. All of our feelings are important and okay to have.

When your child has finished making their feeling characters and heart house, invite them to show you which feeling or feelings are visiting them that day by asking them to put those feeling characters in the heart house. Next, invite them to notice how they feel in their body when each feeling is visiting.

You can support them to say:

(Insert feeling name) is visiting me now.
My body feels like . . . when (*insert feeling name*) is visiting me.

If it is an uncomfortable emotion, you can support them to say:

This is hard for me, or this is a tricky moment.

Then you can support them to say:

All feelings are okay to have. I will feel different soon.

If you feel it is appropriate, you can use the characters and the heart house to show your child the feeling visitors who are visiting your heart that day. You can remind them again that whatever emotion you feel in that moment is okay and that all feelings belong.

WEATHER WHEEL: ACTIVITY 1

Mindfulness helps us to recognize moments when we are struggling, which gives us the opportunity to give ourselves kindness and care. Using the analogy of the weather, this activity supports children to notice times when they are experiencing moments of difficulty. To make this activity, you will need a paper plate, crayons, a split pin, sturdy paper, and scissors. Begin by reflecting with your child about the many different types of weather there can be and invite them to draw the weather types around the outside edge of the paper plate. (Younger children can stick on weather pictures.) The next step is to cut out an arrow shape from the sturdy paper. Then, using the split pin, you can secure the arrow in the middle of the plate, attaching it to the back.

Explain to your child that just like changes in the weather, our feelings and the things that happen in our lives also change. You can tell your child that we can have sunshine times when everything is going well and we feel good inside, cloudy times when life is a bit boring and nothing much is happening, stormy times when life gets a bit difficult, rainy times when we feel a bit down and sad, and rainbow times when we get a beautiful surprise in our lives. Invite your child to think about what other kinds of weather we can have in our lives, and ask them to give some examples. You can share age-appropriate examples of the different types of weather in your life, too.

Using the arrow, invite your child to show you what kind of weather they are having that day. You can remind them that whatever kind of "weather" they are experiencing, that it is okay and it will change again soon.

When your child is experiencing a difficult situation or emotion, you can invite them to show you what kind of weather they are having. You can then support them to say:

Today is an (*insert weather type*) day.
This is hard.
This is a tricky moment.
It is okay to have a day like this and to feel like this.
All my feelings are okay to have.
I will feel different soon.

6

Everyone Has Difficulties

THROUGHOUT MY CAREER, I (Louise) have noticed that so many of us carry deep shame about experiencing difficult situations and emotions. We seem to feel like we have failed or we are "falling short" in some way when we experience times of struggle or difficulty. Due to this sense of falling short, we sometimes tend to hide away during difficult times and not share our struggles or feelings with others, which only escalates our suffering.

Before I began my meditation practice, when I was struggling emotionally I often felt like I must have done something wrong. I would compare myself negatively to others and sometimes felt it was "unfair" that I was suffering and that life was not supposed to be like this. A huge turning point in my life and practice came when I finally understood that I was not "wrong or bad" when I was struggling with difficult situations or emotions and that, instead, this was just a normal part of the experience of being human. I came to understand that my experience of pain or difficulty was, in many ways, nonpersonal.

A nice analogy that illustrates this and the impermanent, impersonal nature of difficult times comes from Jon Kabat-Zinn's "Mountain Meditation." Kabat-Zinn describes that just like the weather changes and the seasons change, we also experience a type of changing seasons in our lives. We experience the summer of life when everything is just wonderful, we are happy, and our children are thriving; autumn, when those good times come to an end and circumstances are changing or challenging; winter, when everything is just difficult, when we or our children are struggling and there doesn't seem to be an end in sight; and spring, when positive changes arrive in our lives and we are filled with hope and inspiration again.

This understanding that suffering is indeed part of the human experience and that nothing I could do would ever change that was like finally taking off a wet, heavy blanket of shame that I had been carrying with me for most of my life. I felt so much lighter. Of course, just like the inevitable changing of the seasons, I still experience difficult times. The difference is that now I don't take these moments so personally. I understand that because I am human, I will have times when I struggle, and that is absolutely okay.

> The very definition of being "human" means that one is mortal, vulnerable, and imperfect. Therefore, self-compassion involves recognizing that suffering and personal inadequacy is part of the shared human experience—something that we all go through rather than being something that happens to "me" alone.
>
> —*Kristin Neff*

Children, too, can experience a huge relief when they learn that they are not alone when encountering difficulty. Just like adults, children may feel embarrassed and sometimes ashamed when they experience difficult situations and uncomfortable emotions. When I am teaching mindfulness in schools, I am often surprised by the number of children who seem to feel shame about having worries and struggles. These children often confide in me that they are too embarrassed to share their concerns with others. They feel that no one else is struggling in the way they are. This sense of isolation can lead to children not sharing their worries with others, which, of course, can create even bigger problems.

When teaching my children's mindfulness classes, the topic of bullying often comes up. Part of the class involves passing around a talking stick where each child has an opportunity to share what is on their mind that day. I remember one particular class when eleven-year-old Sophie (name changed) shared that she was feeling sad because a girl at school was bullying her. When she had finished speaking, a few other children in the group also shared that they, too, had been bullied. The children listened to one another's stories so quietly and intently that you could hear a pin drop in the room.

Afterward, I asked the children who had shared their experiences how it was for them to learn that other kids had similar struggles. I was quite taken aback by the group's response to this question. Sophie said that although she was not happy to learn that the other children had been bullied, it helped her feel less alone. I could really see the relief in the children's faces when they realized that they were not the only ones who had struggled in this way. It was almost like in that moment they were able to let go of some of the shame they had been carrying. There was a real sense of connection, camaraderie, and lightness in the group. It was very touching to witness.

The following activities support children in cultivating an understanding of common humanity by helping them know that they are not alone and that everyone struggles sometimes. When speaking to your child about common humanity, you might like to use the term "noticing others" instead, as this can be much easier for children to say and understand. When sharing these practices with your child, it is important not to minimize their suffering. If your child is struggling, do your best to empathize with them, showing that you really do care about them and the difficulty they are experiencing.

As mentioned previously, although these activities may be very helpful, what is most important is that we do our best to embody a loving, connected presence as we facilitate them with our child. It is also important that we model a sense of common humanity in our everyday lives and interactions with our children. We need to take time to fill our own "cup" with an authentic embodiment of common humanity. As we do this, our children will learn so much about this quality by simply being in our presence.

WORKING WITH STORIES

Common humanity helps us understand that although our outward appearances may be different, human beings are alike in so many ways. This activity supports children in developing an understanding that all people experience difficult emotions and experiences. It also encourages children to cultivate empathy and compassion for others.

To begin, pick an illustrated storybook to read with your child that has a variety of child and adult characters—for example, characters with different ages, nationalities, ethnicities, and so forth. Explain to your child that as you read the story, you will also be taking some time to think and talk about the different characters in the book. As you encounter each new character in the story, pause and reflect together on what is happening for that person.

For example, you could ask your child the following questions about a specific character:

What kind of day do you think this person is having?

What emotion do you think that this person is feeling?

What thoughts do you think this person is thinking?

How do you think they feel in their body?

Do you think this person ever feels sad?

I wonder if this person ever feels worried.

Do you think that this person ever feels angry?

I wonder if this person ever has a hard day.

As your child is answering the questions, practice giving them lots of time and space to express their opinion while you listen to them mindfully and with kindness as best as you can. When they have finished speaking, you can explain that, just like everyone, all of these characters have difficult days sometimes and have times when they feel sad, worried, angry, and afraid.

This activity works best if you support your child to reflect on many different types of characters, ones who range from being similar to being very different from them. It is also advisable to try this exercise with lots of different kinds of books and with characters from movies and TV shows.

WE ARE PART OF THE SAME EARTH

Common humanity teaches us that difficult moments are part of what it means to be human; they are unavoidable, and we are never the only ones who are struggling. This activity will help children understand that they are not alone when they are experiencing an uncomfortable emotion or situation. You will need sturdy paper, crayons and mini people characters for this project.

Have your child cut a large circle out of sturdy paper and tell them that this circle represents the world. Invite them to color in the circle so that it looks like Earth. Next, gather a collection of "mini people" characters—these can be toy miniatures, or your child can make their own "mini people" from cardboard, lollipop sticks, felt, wool, googly eyes, or other craft materials. The characters can represent people from all over the world: children where they live as well as children in other countries they know about—Ireland or Australia, for example. Some could represent children who live in cities or on farms, children in countries they have visited or places they haven't visited, and children from places they have read about or seen on TV.

Show your child the Earth cutout and share with them that there are billions of people in the world. Although these people might look different on the outside and have very different lives, inside, people are alike in many ways. Next, you can share some of the ways that children and people are alike—for example:

People around the world want to be happy.
People around the world have hard days.
People around the world have tricky emotions sometimes.

People around the world make mistakes at times.
People around the world need help sometimes.

Take some time to reflect with your child about other ways people are different and alike. For example, children can look very different on the outside; they can have different-colored hair, skin, and eyes, but inside, all children have similar types of feelings such as anger, sadness, and fear. If your child is having a challenging day or experiencing an uncomfortable emotion, you can take out the Earth cutout and the "mini people" characters. Invite your child to practice "noticing others." Ask them whether they think there is anyone else in the world who is feeling or going through something similar to them. Then help your child to put some characters on the Earth cutout to represent how other children in the world might be experiencing a similar situation or feeling.

You can support your child to softly say to themselves:

So many other children around the world are having a hard time, too.
So many other children around the world are feeling just like me.

MY FAMILY'S FEELINGS

Understanding that all human beings experience difficult emotions can support us to be kinder to ourselves and feel less alone during times of emotional struggle. This activity helps children understand that although the different members of their family may look different on the outside, inside, each family member is similar in many ways. Each person has a heart, and each person experiences a full range of emotions. The activity can also help children develop more compassion and empathy for the other members of their family.

To begin, you can invite your child to draw the outline of themselves and each member of their family on white cardboard. Ask your child to draw a large heart shape on the chest of each person, and then you can help them cut out each of the characters. You can also help them cut around the heart shape so that it opens like a little door while still remaining attached to the person.

Encourage your child to reflect on the different emotions experienced by their family members. You can refer back to the Feeling Friends activity in chapter 5 if you like. You can ask them questions like:

Do you think Dad ever feels sad?
Does Mom ever feel nervous?
Do you know if your brother ever feels shy?
What feelings does your sister have in her heart?

The next step is to stick the characters on a blank sheet of cardboard and invite your child to open up the little heart doors on each of the characters and use different-colored crayons to represent the feelings inside each person's heart. Invite them to decorate each of the characters and the background.

When the picture is finished, help your child to open and close the little heart doors. Encourage them to notice that although each family member looks different on the outside, when we look inside their heart, each person is very alike and has just the same kind of feelings.

You can support your child to say:

Outside, we might look different; inside, we are just the same.

WEATHER WHEEL: ACTIVITY 2

Common humanity teaches us that just like challenging weather is part of life, difficult situations and uncomfortable emotions are part of life, too. The practice also shows us that just like challenging weather is impersonal, experiencing difficult situations and emotions is also, in many ways, impersonal. It is simply part of what it means to be a human being.

This activity helps children to recognize that simply because we are alive, we will sometimes experience moments of struggle and uncomfortable emotions. It also teaches children that just like the weather is always changing, our emotions and the circumstances of our lives are also always changing and that no matter what happens in our lives or however we feel, we can always be kind to ourselves.

This activity uses the same "weather wheel" introduced in Weather Wheel: Activity 1 in chapter 5. You can find instructions on how to make the weather wheel there. Share with your child that just like it is not our fault when it is raining or stormy, it is also not our fault when we are finding life hard or having uncomfortable emotions. Just like rainy, cloudy, and stormy weather conditions are part of life, going through hard times and struggling with our emotions are sometimes part of life, too. Take out the prepared weather wheel and, using the arrow, invite your child to show you what kind of weather they are having that day. It can be helpful if you show your child the type of weather that you are experiencing, if you feel it is appropriate. You can remind them that whatever kind of "weather" they are experiencing today, that's okay. It will change soon. Whatever the weather, we can always practice being kind to ourselves.

You can support your child to say kindly to themself:

Hard moments are part of life.
Everyone has hard moments sometimes.
Tricky emotions are part of life.
Everyone has tricky emotions sometimes.

"HAVE THEY EVER . . ." BASKET

You can use a basket and little stuffed animals for this visual and interactive activity to help children understand that everyone struggles sometimes. Have enough stuffed animals available to use for each family member, as well as some extras. The extras can be used to represent other people in your child's life, such as friends or relatives. They can also represent groups of people—for example, one for kids at school, on their team, in their gymnastics class, in the neighborhood; one for their friends, one for children they sometimes find difficult, one for children they do not know, one for grown-ups they know, and one for grown-ups they don't know.

Now, starting with one example of experiencing difficulty from the list below or coming up with your own, pick up a stuffed animal and say, "I wonder if other children at school (for example) have ever made a mistake (for example)."

This is a gentle inquiry where you support them in seeing that even if it is a different mistake than the one they have made, everyone makes mistakes at times. Sometimes it can help to use yourself as the first stuffed animal, reassuring them that you have made mistakes. As you acknowledge this, have your child put that stuffed animal in the basket. Now, pick up another stuffed animal to represent someone else and continue asking if they can imagine if that person has ever made a mistake. Continue by using the other stuffed animals to represent other people or groups of people who may also have made a mistake. This visual activity is a way to engage in conversation about common humanity: everyone has things that are hard for them, and everyone struggles at times.

You can go through the same process with other difficulties listed below or focus on just one that they may be struggling with at the time. This basket with stuffed animals can serve as a visual reminder of common humanity and can be kept in their special space. If they are dealing with something difficult, you can take it out. It can be used to remind them that of course they are feeling the way they are. Everyone has a hard time sometimes.

The following are some ideas to use with this activity:

Made a mistake
Had a hard time at school
Had their feelings hurt
Felt nervous doing something new
Felt grouchy about something
Felt unkind
Felt embarrassed about something they did or said
Wasn't included
Was lonely
Needed help

Felt overwhelmed

Didn't do as well as they would have liked (on a test, an activity, a
sport . . .)

"JUST LIKE ME" MEDITATION

In chapters 2 and 3, we introduced practices to cultivate a sense of common humanity for adults: Just Like Me, How Human of Me and I Am Not the Only One. This meditation is an adaptation for children of the Just Like Me practice.

The following meditation may be helpful to practice with your child when they experience moments of struggle or uncomfortable feelings. You can invite them to sit or lie down as they listen to the meditation— whichever they feel most comfortable with. You also might like to put on some gentle music in the background.

"JUST LIKE ME" MEDITATION SCRIPT

If you like, you can close your eyes and begin to notice your breathing. Can you notice your breathing in and breathing out? What does it feel like to just notice your breathing in and breathing out for a little while?

Now, we are going to use our imagination.

Can you imagine your family standing in a circle all around you? Have a look into their eyes and give them a little smile if you like. Do you know that just like you, your family wants to feel happy? Do you know that just like you, every member of your family has hard moments sometimes and feels tricky feelings, too?

You can say to yourself:

Just like me, my family wants to be happy. Just like me, my family
has hard moments sometimes and feels tricky feelings, too.

Now, can you imagine your friends standing in a circle all around you? Look into their eyes and give them a little smile if you like. Do you know that just like you, your friends want to be happy? And just like you, your friends have hard moments sometimes and feel tricky feelings, too.

You can say to yourself:

Just like me, my friends want to be happy. Just like me, my friends have hard moments sometimes and feel tricky feelings, too.

Imagine all of the children in your class standing around you. Notice what they look like and give them a little smile if you like. Just like you, all of the children in your class want to be happy. And just like you, they all have hard moments sometimes and feel tricky feelings, too.

Now, you can say to yourself:

Just like me, the children in my class want to be happy. Just like me, they all have hard moments sometimes and feel tricky feelings, too.

Can you imagine all the people you know around you? Give them a little smile if you like. Do you know that just like you, all of the people you know want to be happy? And just like you, all of the people you know have hard moments sometimes and feel tricky feelings, too.

You can say to yourself:

Just like me, all of the people I know want to be happy. Just like me, all of the people I know have hard moments sometimes and feel tricky feelings, too.

Can you notice your breath again? Can you notice how you feel inside? How does your head feel? How does your body feel? How does your heart feel? Remember, however you feel right now, that's okay. It is always okay to feel like you do. When you are ready, you can wriggle your fingers and toes and open your eyes.

7

Befriending Ourselves
in Difficult Moments

SOMETHING THAT I (LOUISE) hear consistently from the adults I work with is how they wish someone had taught them about the importance of being kinder to themselves when they were younger. They often wonder how different their life would have been. I genuinely believe that one of the most important things that we can teach our children is to be kind to themselves. In my experience, this is one of the greatest ways we support them to lead happy, healthy, and fulfilling lives.

Self-kindness encompasses a sense of our inherent value. We recognize that we have value and are worthy of love, care, and compassion simply because we exist. Our value does not depend on our personal achievements, outward appearance, or how well we are doing in life.

I like to describe self-kindness as nurturing a genuine and loving friendship with ourselves. It is offering ourselves the same kindness and care that we would give to a best friend, and it is knowing that we are always deeply deserving of this care and compassion. With mindfulness practice, we cultivate intimacy with ourselves, we meet ourselves as we are. With self-kindness, we bring an attitude of care, compassion, and love to ourselves, wrapping ourselves up in that warm blanket of kindness.

Throughout my career, I have found that when children learn to be authentically kind to themselves, they will be more likely to take care of themselves well, less likely to engage in activities that could be harmful to themselves or others, and less inclined to accept unkind treatment from others. They will also tend to have an innate understanding of their own worth and inner goodness, which leads to them honoring themselves more and cultivating healthier and more positive relationships with others.

Part of my work involves visiting schools to share the practices of mindfulness and self-compassion with children. Something that I notice, on a consistent basis, is that very few children have any understanding of how to be kind to themselves or what that even means. Children are often taught about being kind to others, but it seems that they are rarely encouraged to be kind to themselves.

I also notice that as children get older, they struggle more with practicing kindness toward themselves. While four- and five-year-olds tend to find it relatively easy and fun to name one thing they like about themselves, eleven- and twelve-year-olds may find this same task deeply embarrassing and often refuse to do it. This saddens me. However, it also serves as an inspiration to share this work with as many children and families as possible. The wonderful thing is that just like we can teach children their letters and numbers and about geography and history, we can also teach them how to be a caring friend to themselves, to offer themselves kindness during moments of difficulty, and to recognize their own intrinsic worth and value.

The next section introduces some activities that I have found particularly helpful in sharing self-kindness with children. Remember that the greatest gift we can give children is our loving, compassionate presence. It will be a huge support to our children if we can embody this compassionate presence as much as we can as we facilitate these activities and, of course, in our daily interactions with them.

INNER KIND FRIEND

In my work with children, I always share that it is just as important to be kind to ourselves as it is to be kind to others. I explain that being kind to ourselves is like being our own best friend and that we can speak to ourselves and treat ourselves the way a best friend might speak to or treat us.

To begin, invite your child to imagine the kindest, most caring, most loving friend. Encourage them to picture their friend in great detail. What sort of eyes do they have? What is their voice like? What might their gestures be? What else can you notice about them? (You can use the Kind Friend Reflection practice on the following page if you'd like.)

Ask your child to think of the words their kind friend might say to them and then practice saying these kind words to themselves. You can support them to write out these words on pieces of paper and put them in a little bag or envelope. For younger children, you can write the words for them to read together later. They can also draw pictures to put in the bag. To make this activity more interactive, invite your child to make their inner friend. This can be as simple as drawing the kind friend on paper and coloring it in; or it can be made with clay, material, wool, cardboard, googly eyes, or any other craft bits that you have.

The kind friend can also be a doll, teddy, or toy character. When your child is experiencing a difficult emotion or situation, invite them to take out their kind friend and read the caring messages they carry in their bag, or support them to think about what words their friend might say to them and what advice they might give them.

A way to extend this activity, particularly when your child is experiencing difficulty, is for them to write a letter to themselves from the perspective of their kind friend. The letter might contain some caring words and some suggestions on ways they could be kind and caring to themselves. Depending on the age of your child, you might need to support them with this. Younger children might want to draw on or stick pictures to the letter.

KIND FRIEND REFLECTION

You can close your eyes, if you feel comfortable, and take a nice deep breath in and out.

Now, we are going to use our imagination. Can you imagine the kindest, most loving, most caring friend you can think of? This friend can be a person, an animal, a magical creature, or anything that you can imagine. The most important thing is that this friend is so kind and so caring. They love you so much, they understand you, and they want to be there for you and to help you.

Can you take a really close look at your kind friend? What sort of eyes do they have? What type of voice does your friend have?

What sort of words do they say?

Do you know you can ask your kind friend a question or tell them about something that is bothering you? Their words are so loving, caring, and wise.

Is there anything you would like to ask your kind friend or anything you would like to tell them? Do they have any messages for you?

How do you feel inside after spending some time with your kind friend? How does your head, body, and heart feel? Remember, however you feel inside right now, that's okay. It's okay to feel like you do.

If you like, you can take a little time to relax with your kind friend, and then when you are ready, you can wriggle your fingers and toes, have a big stretch, and open your eyes.

Remember, it is important to also always tell a grown-up you trust about any worries you may have or anything that is upsetting you.

THE KINDNESS KINGDOM

The Kindness Kingdom practice is an expansion of the Kind Friend Reflection activity and is a great way to help children cultivate the full spectrum of self-compassionate qualities from "softer" qualities to stronger, more action-based qualities.

Begin by inviting your child to imagine a beautiful, magical kingdom and explain to them that all of the creatures who live in this kingdom are very kind, caring, and loving.

The characters could be elves, fairies, princes and princesses, animals, or any other creature your child can imagine. The inhabitants of the "Kingdom of Kindness" can range from very gentle and soft characters to much stronger, protecting, and motivating characters.

You can help your child imagine what the personalities of the different "kindness creatures" might be like. What might they look like? What type of voice might they have? What would their tone of voice be like? What sort of words might they use? What gestures might they use? What would they suggest your child do? (You can use the Kind Friend Reflection here if you'd like.)

You can invite your child to make their own Kingdom of Kindness, where all of their kind friends live. The Kingdom of Kindness can be made using empty boxes stuck together. Children can decorate the front of the boxes to represent a castle and make little paper turrets to stick on top of the boxes. Over time, you can help your child create the different characters who live in their Kingdom of Kindness. The characters can be made from clay, cardboard, stones, wooden pegs, felt, or other materials. They can also just be stuffed animals or dolls belonging to your child.

This is an activity that you and your child can really play with. Children can create stories and act out little scenarios with the creatures. When your child is having a tough day or is experiencing an uncomfortable emotion, invite them to imagine which kind creature might be good to ask for some help. They can imagine what advice their kind creature might give and what words they might say. They can also imagine what their tone of voice and gestures might be. You can encourage your child to practice being like this kind friend to themselves. As they offer themselves words and gestures of kindness, invite them to notice how they feel inside their heart, mind, and body.

Your child can also write letters and notes and create drawings to and from the different characters in the Kindness Kingdom. Depending on the age of your child, you might need to support them with this.

CUP OF SUNSHINE

Another activity that can help children cultivate kindness toward themselves is the Cup of Sunshine activity. The "cup of sunshine" represents their cup of happiness and well-being. This activity teaches children about the importance of taking care of themselves and how looking after themselves well positively impacts their emotions and how they feel in their bodies.

This can be done by drawing a cup on a sheet of paper; however, I find it works best using a paper cup. You can encourage your child to think about all the ways that they can be kind and caring to themselves, from "softer" practices, such as putting their hand on their heart, to "stronger" ways, like asking for help with something or moving their body. Children can write or draw pictures of these acts of self-kindness and then put them in their cup. You can use small picture cutouts for younger children. An important part of this activity is to help children reflect on what it feels like inside their bodies when they do the things that fill up their cup of sunshine. Invite each child to reflect on how their mind, body, and heart feel when their cup of sunshine is full in comparison to when it's empty.

It works really well if you can make your own cup of sunshine and share authentically with your child as you both make and fill your cups of sunshine together. If they are having a difficult time, take out the cup of sunshine and invite them to think about what they could do to fill up their cup a little more today.

Each evening or every so often, you and your child can take out your cups of sunshine and talk about one way you filled your cup that day. You can also invite them to think about how they might fill their cup of sunshine the next day.

You might also like to reflect on the following questions with your child:

How full was your cup of sunshine today?
How does it feel in your body when your cup of sunshine is full?

How does it feel in your body when your cup of sunshine is empty?
What is your favorite way to fill your cup of sunshine?
I wonder how we can help fill other people's cups of sunshine?

HEART CONTAINER

Self-kindness can be described as a kind attitude toward the self in painful moments rather than harsh self-criticism and self-degradation. This activity is another way to use the heart container from the Hold It in a Loving Heart practice presented in chapter 4. It supports children in cultivating a kind and loving attitude toward themselves when they are experiencing uncomfortable emotions. This activity focuses on children's relationship with their emotions and the attitude they bring to themselves as the "experiencer" of those emotions.

You can use the heart container you made in chapter 4, or use clay to make a container, which can be heart shaped or any shape your child likes. Explain to your child that this container represents their heart. Once your child has made their heart container, you can invite them to make their feelings using little balls of clay and share that you are also going to make some feelings to put inside the heart. Children can then paint their container and let it dry and paint and draw faces on the clay balls to represent their different emotions.

When the container is dry, you can invite your child to think about some kind words that they could say to their feelings. You can also ask older children to imagine if their heart could talk to their feelings, what kind words it would say to them. You can experiment with this together by holding the feelings in your hands and imagining some caring words you can say to them. When your child has thought of some kind words to say to their feelings, you can help them write these messages of kindness on the container (paint markers work well for this). For example, if your child was feeling sad about not being invited to a party, you could support them to hold their "sad feeling" gently in their hands and to say kind words to it. They could say, "I am here for you," or "I will look after you."

Like the other creative activities, this practice works best when the heart container is interacted with regularly. The container can be used to help children identify and communicate which feelings they are experiencing. Children can put the emotion, or emotions, that they are experiencing in the container and then practice saying the words on the container to their feelings. Younger children may need extra support with this. Practicing this along with your child using your own heart container and feelings will greatly support your child with this activity.

I AM A SHINING STAR

When we are truly kind to ourselves, we recognize that our worth is not dependent on our external achievements, successes, or outward appearance. Instead, we have an understanding that we have value and worth simply because we are "us," simply because we exist. One way to teach children about their own and others' intrinsic value is the I Am a Shining Star activity. You can begin by giving your child a small star shape cut out of gold-colored sturdy paper. I like to put the star in a small drawstring bag.

Tell your child that they are just like a "shining star," and share that there is no one in the world any better than them, no one in the world any less than them, no one in the world the same as them. They are unique and precious, just like a shining star.

Explain that every other child is like a shining star, too. Just like a shining star, every child is unique, and each child in the world has equal value and is equally important. Tell your child that they are precious and important simply because they are themselves and that no matter what happens in life, they will always be this shining star.

This activity can be particularly effective when you notice your child comparing themselves to others or feeling like they are inadequate in some way. Invite them to hold the star in their hands. Again, explain to them that there is no child in the world who is better than them and no child in the world who is less than them; that they are unique and precious, just like a shining star. Then share that in order to shine brightly like a star in the world, they need to do three things:

1. Be kind to themselves.
2. Be kind to others.
3. Just try their best.

Explain that they never need to be the best, but it is important that they try their best. Now invite your child to give themselves a big hug and say to themselves, "I am a shining star." The star can be kept in a little drawstring bag in your child's special space, or they could even keep it in their pocket or schoolbag on a day they might need a little extra support.

A nice way to extend this activity is to invite them to trace their finger around the star shape. Starting at the top of the star, ask your child to take a deep breath in as they trace the inward sides of the star and then take a slow breath out as they trace the outward sides. You can also invite your child to say an affirmation or one thing they like about themselves as they reach each of the star's five points.

Affirmation suggestions:

I am loved.
I am safe.
I am just right.
I am a good friend.
I shine just like a star.

"YOU ARE LOVED" BOOK

When children know that they are deeply cared about and valued for exactly who they are, they will be supported to cultivate more kindness and care for themselves and to integrate a deeper sense of self-worth and intrinsic value. The "You Are Loved" Book is a helpful activity that will encourage children to really take in the love and care of family members and loved ones.

You will need an empty scrapbook for this activity. Begin by giving the scrapbook to family members and friends with whom your child has a close connection. Invite each person to stick a picture of themselves—preferably a picture of themselves with your child—on a blank page of the scrapbook. Then invite each person to write underneath the picture three things that they love or admire about your child. They can also include a happy memory they have with your child or an activity they like to do with them. For example, Grandma might write, "I love that you are kind, I love that you are funny, I love that you make me laugh, I really enjoy reading books with you."

When the "You Are Loved" Book is complete, take some time to read through the pages together with your child. You can reflect back to them the caring words on each page—for example, "Grandma loves you so much; she thinks you are funny and thoughtful, and she loves reading stories with you." Encourage your child to notice how they feel inside their body when they read the kind words each person said about them. They can also put their hand on their heart and say the kind words out loud as affirmations—for example, "I am kind, I am funny, Grandma loves me so much." Then invite your child to give themselves a big hug.

When your child is having a difficult day, you can take out the book and read it together. After reading through the book together, you can support them to notice how much they are loved and valued by all of the wonderful people in their life. Then you can invite your child to see if they can practice being caring and loving to themselves. Ask them to think of some kind words they can say to themselves and some caring things that they can do for themselves.

If you would like to extend this activity, you can practice the following "I Am Loved" Reflection with your child.

"I AM LOVED" REFLECTION

If you like, you can close your eyes and take a nice deep breath in and out.

Can you think about some of the people in your life who make you feel the most loved and cared for? It could be a parent, grandparent, aunt, uncle, friend, or someone else.

Imagine these people standing in a circle all around you. Take some time to really notice each person.

What do you like about these people?

Think of some happy memories with them.

How does it feel inside when you are with these people?

Can you think of how much all of these people love and care for you? They love you so much!

Can you imagine the love from their hearts is like golden, sparkling sunshine? Imagine this beautiful sunshine is all around you. Beautiful, bright sunshine swirling, twirling, and twinkling all around you.

Now put both your hands on your heart if you like, take a big deep breath in, and breathe in this beautiful sunshine. Breathe this sparkling sunshine into your heart.

You can say to yourself, "I am loved."

Keep breathing in this sunshine filled with love into your heart.

Imagine your heart filled up with this sparkling, shining love.

Feel your hand on your heart, and say to yourself, "I am cared for."

Feel this shining sunshine fill up every part of your body, from the top of your head to the tips of your toes. See yourself completely filled up with this warm, twinkling sunshine, filled with love.

Feel your hands filled up with this sunshine, and feel the sunshine stream through your hands toward your heart.

Say to yourself: "I love and care for myself. I am a good friend to myself."

Now, if you like, breathe out some of this shining sunshine filled with love to the people around you who love and care for you.

As you breathe out the sunshine, see them smile. Now make a kind wish for them if you like.

May you be safe and healthy.

May you be happy and peaceful.

Thank these people for being kind and caring to you, and keep breathing in and out the shining sunshine filled with love.

Breathe in sparkling sunshine for you.

Breathe out this loving sunshine for others.

In for you.

Out for others.

Can you notice how you feel now? How does your head, heart, and body feel? Remember, however you feel, that's okay. It's okay to feel like you do.

Wriggle your fingers and toes, have a big stretch, then slowly open your eyes.

8

Embodied Self-Awareness and Self-Compassion

THROUGHOUT THIS BOOK, and as a part of multiple practices, we have encouraged cueing your child to notice how their body is feeling. Here we will dive more deeply into supporting children to be increasingly embodied as they go about their lives. We want to help them notice how their body feels when things are hard and how to support themselves by embodying self-compassion. Feeling the difficult experiences and knowing how to best look after ourselves in those moments, as well as feeling pleasant experiences and knowing how to let them sink in, is an essential skill for ongoing well-being. Caring for ourselves includes caring for our nervous system, which begins with getting to know it better through body awareness.

We live our lives in these bodies, and they are constantly sending us information. Often it is in the body that we get the first signal to notice our emotional weather, to use the mindfulness metaphor from chapter 5. In this way, deepening our somatic, felt physical awareness supports our mindfulness practice. Because it is such a crucial component of self-awareness and mindfulness, when teaching children, I (Wendy) do multiple activities to focus on how emotions are experienced in our bodies.

You can integrate body awareness into everyday life by periodically asking children to notice how their body feels. For example, encourage them to notice how it feels when they are being silly, playing with friends, doing some physical activity, singing, dancing, walking in nature, or even sitting quietly. Some children who are really in touch with their bodily sensations will find this easier to do, like the child in one of my classes who described his head feeling "tight" and "crunchy" when he was frustrated. However, some children may initially need support. If so, it can help to offer them some ideas, such as asking if they notice how their belly or shoulders feel. You could ask if they notice a lot of energy in their body; or if it feels hard or soft, tight or loose. It is important to remind children that whatever they feel, it is always okay. It can be helpful if you also share with them how your body feels at different times. For example, after a long day, you might share that you notice your body doesn't have a lot of energy or that you notice a heavy sensation in your head.

FEELING SENSATION CARDS

The Feeling Sensation Cards activity expands on increasing children's body awareness, especially as it relates to big emotions. Begin by giving examples of different things that may cause strong emotions, such as having lots of homework, not being included with others at recess, having fun plans get canceled, or not getting a part in a school play. Use scenarios that you feel your child can relate to. Now ask them to notice how it feels in their body when they imagine these situations.

Again, it can be hard for children (and adults) to identify body sensations, and it is sometimes helpful to cue them specifically toward different body parts and give examples, as mentioned in the beginning of the chapter. You might say, "How did your belly or your heart feel when you found out about the surprise quiz?" In my work with children, I also find that they will often use "emotion words" to say how their body feels. For example, they may say their body "feels worried" and not identify the actual sensations they experience. When that happens, you might say, "I'm wondering how the emotion of being worried feels in your body. How does your belly feel?" If they can't identify the sensation, you could also say, "Maybe your belly felt all swirly when you found out about the surprise quiz." As appropriate, you can also share your emotions and the sensations you notice, such as, "When our fun plans were canceled the other day, I was sad and my heart felt heavy." Here you are naming both the emotion and the connected physical sensation.

Next, talk about what images might remind them of those sensations. Some of the following examples can help: fire for hot, knots for tight, weights for heavy, feathers for light, a tornado for swirling, or a lightning bolt for energy. Of course, as they want to, let them come up with their own ideas. For some children, tapping into their creativity helps them get more curious about how emotions feel in their bodies. Write down a list of the different sensations and corresponding images you identified together.

To make the cards, cut rectangles out of sturdy paper. Write the name of one sensation from your list on the top of each card. Then your child can draw and color an image to represent that sensation, or you could stick an image onto the card. To make them extra sturdy, the cards can be laminated. If you like, you can put Velcro on the back of the cards so they can be stuck to clothes or stuffed animals.

Use the cards in discussions about how emotions feel in the body. For example, you could put the knot card on your belly to show how you feel when you are worried. You can then ask your child to use the cards and show how parts of their body feel in different situations or when they are experiencing a particular emotion. This can be especially helpful if they are sharing a story about something or are in the midst of a strong emotion. Identifying and experiencing sensations can help slow things down and decrease the momentum of an emotion.

Your child can also put a card on a buddy—a stuffed animal—to show how they or their buddy might feel. For example, they may put a "heavy sensation" card on their buddy's heart to show you how they felt at school when no one would play with them. You can also use the buddy to say, "I wonder how your buddy's heart would feel if it had no one to play with?" If they don't have any ideas, the cards can be used to give some examples. You could wonder together if it might feel heavy, tight, or swirly. Give them many options, and always remind them that there are no right or wrong answers. However they feel is always okay.

LUGGAGE FOR OUR FEELING VISITORS

You can also expand on the Feeling Sensation Cards (above) and Heart House and Feeling Visitors (chap. 5) activities. For this activity, you will need some small drawstring bags, cards, and markers. Take out the previously made heart house and feeling visitors, as well as the feeling sensation cards from above. Tell your child that when our feelings come to visit us, they also bring some luggage with them. Explain that the luggage is the different sensations we feel in our body when we are having that emotion. Now put one of the emotion characters in the heart house and invite your child to share how they feel in their body when this emotion comes to visit. Using the feeling sensation cards, your child can show you where in their body they feel those sensations. You and your child can repeat this process for each of their feeling visitors. Remind your child that all feelings and sensations are okay to have; the most important thing is that we look after ourselves well and are kind to ourselves when our feelings come to visit.

The next step is to give your child a small drawstring bag (luggage) for each of their feeling visitors and then ask them to make mini sensation cards to represent the bodily sensations each feeling brings with them. The mini sensations cards are made in the same way as in the previous activity but need to be small enough to fit in the bags. When the cards are made, invite your child to put them in the corresponding feeling visitor's bag. The feeling sensation cards, feeling visitors, and luggage can all be particularly helpful tools to use in any activity where we suggest you support your child in noticing how they feel inside.

PARADE OF EMOTIONS

One of my favorite activities to do with children stems from a game I used to play with my own children when they were little and was the inspiration for my book *The Monster Parade*. The parade analogy reminds us that our emotions, as well as the physical sensations that go along with them, are just passing by, and yet they are in a parade and want our attention. This can be a helpful reminder, especially with unpleasant or uncomfortable emotions and physical sensations.

Have your child or group of children imagine they are in a parade. Clarify a few rules before you begin, especially in a large group. For example, decide on the parade route, explain that the characters in the parade do not touch each other, and decide whether or not they make noises based on your preference. Include any other rules you feel would be helpful before beginning the game. Let them know you will be using a bell to freeze the parade. Explain that when you ring the bell, they should freeze as the parade characters. Alternatively, you can have them move to music as the parade characters, and when you stop the music, they freeze.

Give them a scenario that may illicit a big emotion. For example, have them parade like someone who is going to a new school, just scored in the big game, had to clean their room instead of doing something fun, was just playing and laughing with friends, is having a hard time with their schoolwork, or whose best friend is moving. You can use scenarios that you feel may resonate with your child.

When you ring the bell (or stop the music), ask them to notice how their body feels after parading like the person in this situation. Can they name the emotion and say how it feels in their body? Another option is just to say an emotion and have them parade in that way, focusing on the felt sensory experience of the emotion. You can also have them parade in fun and silly ways, such as like a king or queen, a bird, or the wind; like they are walking on thin ice or sneaking up on someone. Again, when they freeze, talk about how it feels in their body to be these things. As you discuss this activity, you are helping your child understand the relationship between their body and their emotions.

You can also integrate the feeling sensation cards into this activity by making the cards in the shape of balloons and asking what balloons they are carrying in the parade when they feel different emotions. For example, if they feel sad, maybe they are carrying the heavy balloon, or the fuzzy balloon if their brain feels a bit fuzzy, or the turtle balloon if they feel slow and low-energy. Follow their lead, giving them space to be creative in expressing how emotions are felt in their body, and always remind them that all their feelings and sensations are welcome in the parade.

Embodied Practices Can Help in Difficult Moments

As we have seen, by connecting with the experience in our bodies, we can better understand our emotions. We can also use body-based practices to support ourselves in difficult moments. These embodied practices have physiological and emotional benefits, which can make a difference when things are hard. The better we understand the connection between our bodies and our moods, the more skillful we can be in accessing our bodies to heal our hearts and minds and teach our children to do so as well.

Learning many ways that my body can help shift my mood has made such a difference in my life. Whether it be dancing around the house, going for a walk in the woods, practicing some yoga, having a cup of tea (and noticing the warm, soothing sensation), or offering myself kind touch, these practices have all been tremendously beneficial. Through embodied practices, we can help our children develop this powerful life-changing capacity for self-care and well-being.

The Gift of Kind Touch

Those who know me are not surprised to hear me teach about the practice of putting your hand on your heart. This is something I have done for many years. Long before I learned that it was in fact a "practice," I instinctively offered myself kindness in this way to soothe my nervous system. When I do, I have this sense of being held and connected. It is an act of love and coming home to myself.

This kind touch, which we practiced in chapter 2, is one helpful way of physically caring for ourselves. It both feels good and is good for us. When we gently touch ourselves as an offering of kindness and care, it releases oxytocin. This feel-good hormone supports a felt sense of connection and downregulates our nervous system activation as it brings the care system online.[13] When I feel moved by someone else's struggles, a hand on the heart has been my way of saying my heart is here for you. How lovely when we can also say that to ourselves in this embodied way.

KIND TOUCH PRACTICES FOR CHILDREN

As we did in chapter 2 for ourselves, we can help our children learn to offer themselves this "kind touch." Have your child try the different types of touch that are listed in that activity and ask them to notice how each feels for them. Have them imagine their hand is filled with warmth and love as they take in the offering of care to and from themselves. Another option is to have them imagine it is a loved one offering this kindness to them, especially if it is hard to offer it to themselves.

Learning to give themselves a hug, one of the many ways to offer kind touch, can be particularly helpful for children who struggle when separating from their parents. I remind them that when they give themselves a hug, they can pretend that the adult they miss is hugging them. In my experience, many children find it helpful to begin by offering themselves kind touch while thinking of someone who loves them as they learn to internalize it as a way to offer love to themselves.

You can play with adding words to the Kind Touch practice. Though we will explore this more in the next chapter, it can be helpful to integrate an embodied aspect into the practice of offering yourself words of kindness and care. Encourage children to stop and notice how it feels in their body when they offer themselves kind touch and say to themselves, "I am here for you," or "You've got this," or "I love you."

SELF-COMPASSION BLANKET

At the beginning of the book, I shared about my friend who encouraged me to imagine that her love for me was like a warm and cozy blanket. This felt sense of love and care is powerful and can bring us the comfort we need in difficult moments. We can use our imagination, as I did at that time, to experience kindness and warmth coming from someone else while actually offering it to ourselves.

You and your child can begin by choosing a blanket to be used specifically for this practice. Sit together with the blanket in your arms, and take a few gentle breaths as you both settle in. Ask your child to imagine that you are filling up the blanket with your love for them. They could picture light and warmth going from you into the blanket. They may even want to close their eyes for a moment to imagine this more clearly. You can wait a few seconds to let that image sink in. Then ask them to open their eyes again as you give the blanket a hug, putting your hugs, love, and caring into the blanket before handing it over to them. This self-compassion blanket, or blanket of love, is now ready to use, and if they want, they can put it in their special space. When they are having a difficult time, they can physically experience the love and care they need by wrapping themselves in this self-compassion blanket.

You can take this practice one step further by using the props from the Feeling Visitors and the Feeling Sensation Cards activities, with an actual blanket. This aspect of the practice is adapted from an activity in the Self-Compassion for Children and Caregivers program designed by Jamie Lynn Tatera. You can discuss what emotion might be visiting and what sensations accompany that emotion, as we did in the previous activities. Now have your child take the relevant feeling visitors and feeling sensation cards and wrap them in the blanket as you talk about how we can also wrap our emotions and sensations in our self-compassion blanket. In this way, we further embody the message that when we have big emotions and sensations that may feel uncomfortable, we can also offer them love, comfort, and care. Self-compassion, in the form of our blanket, can hold us and all of our uncomfortable emotions and sensations.

The child can stay wrapped, feeling comforted and cozy in the blanket, while using the edges of the blanket to practice wrapping the emotions and sensations in this way. You can guide them to say something supportive, like "I can wrap myself, this sadness, and the feeling of heaviness inside with lots of love and kindness." You can assure your child that no matter what emotion or sensation they feel, they are all okay to feel, and they all can be wrapped in kindness and love.

SELF-COMPASSION BLANKET VISUALIZATION

The following practice can support children internalizing a felt sense of the self-compassion blanket without having an actual blanket. Doing this practice periodically will help your child so they can access this feeling of love and care in a moment of need.

SELF-COMPASSION BLANKET VISUALIZATION SCRIPT

Close your eyes if you like, and take a few gentle breaths in and out.

Now imagine that I am giving you a comfy, cozy, imaginary blanket and that this special blanket is filled with my love for you. The love could be like sparkles or twinkling light, or it could be a solid color that fills up the blanket with so much love.

Can you look closely to see what your special blanket looks like?

What color is it?

Is it shimmering and sparkling, or is it solid?

How big is it?

What is it made out of?

How soft is it? Maybe it is smooth and silky or soft and puffy?

Is it light or heavy?

See if you can notice what it feels like to hold it.

Now imagine you are being wrapped up in this blanket of love and care in any way that feels just right for you. Maybe loosely over your shoulders, all bundled up tight and cozy, or any way that is good for you.

How does it feel to be wrapped up in this blanket filled with love and kindness?

Remember, the blanket is in your imagination, so it is here for you always, just like my love is here for you always, holding you with warmth and so much kindness.

Especially if things feel hard, you can wrap yourself up in this blanket of love.

You can always count on your blanket to help you be kind to yourself and remind yourself that it is always here for you. You just have to remember to use it.

You might even think to yourself, "This is my special blanket of kindness and love," as you feel it wrapping you up like a warm and cozy hug.

(Pause for three to five breaths.)

Can you notice how you feel now? How does your body feel? How does your head feel? How does your heart feel? Remember, however you feel, that's okay. All of your feelings are okay to have.

And now, as you are ready, slowly and gently move your body, wriggle your fingers and your toes, and gently open your eyes if they were closed.

YOGA

Practicing yoga with your child can help them understand and work with the interconnection of the body and emotions. When I teach yoga to children and adults, I often focus on noticing the impact of postures on our emotions, mind states, and other bodily sensations. I encourage noticing things like changes in energy, feeling tight or loose, or noticing the body feeling big like the sky or even "crunchy," as the previously mentioned child told me he felt when dealing with frustration.

There are many yoga resources for children. I recommend using resources that encourage children to notice how their body feels and to check in on any changes in energy and emotions.

You can try a few of these ideas as well. I encourage you to do these poses along with your child so you can feel the impact of them as you discuss them with your child. Be curious and invite your child to be curious about how it feels physically and emotionally when doing the following poses.

SEATED MOUNTAIN: Sit like you are a mountain, either on a chair, possibly with your feet on the ground, or on the floor in a way that feels like a mountain to you. Can you notice what parts of your body change or shift? Maybe your shoulders drop down, your back lifts up a bit; maybe your head shifts position and your legs and belly tighten a bit more. Maybe you feel strong and steady or possibly heavy and tight. Whatever you notice is always okay and is true for you. The ideas listed here are just offered as examples, not expectations of how you should feel. Invite your child to scan their body and be curious about what they notice.

TREE: Stand like a tree, rooted through both feet or in a traditional yoga Tree Pose with one leg bent at the knee and turned out to the side and the foot either resting by the ankle or higher up on the leg. You can lift your arms up into the air in whatever way feels good to you. In our practice, we are not trying to achieve any particular look for the pose. Instead, we are noticing the connection between the postures and how we feel inside. Imagine that your body is the trunk of the tree, your arms are the branches, and your feet are the roots going down deeply into the ground. Notice how Tree Pose feels in your body and any impact it may have on your emotions.

WARRIOR: Place one foot a few feet in front of the other and bend the knee of the front leg. Raise your arms up in a strong V shape. Notice the strength in your legs and arms. I often use an affirmation when I teach this pose. You could count to three and then say together, "I can do it," then bend your arms with fists coming to your chest and make a loud *ha* sound. How does that feel in your heart and body? Do you feel strong and steady in this pose? Again, there are no right or wrong answers. Whatever you notice is always okay.

BREATH OF JOY: Stand with your feet hip-width apart and your knees slightly bent. I often tell children, with this more active posture, to imagine their feet are glued to the ground to support some stability. Swing your arms in front of you, swing them behind you, and then swing them up to the sky. Finally, swing them behind you again as you bend your knees and release down at your hips for a forward bend as you make a loud *ha* sound. Do a few Breaths of Joy and then stop and notice how your body is feeling, including any shift in energy or mood.

RAG DOLL: Stand with your feet close together with a slight bend at your knees. Again, with this posture I suggest telling your child to imagine their feet are glued to the ground. Now bend from your hips, going into a forward bend. Invite the upper part of your body to be loose and soft. You can even play with swaying your body back and forth like a rag doll with the reminder that the feet stay connected to the ground at all times. As with the other postures, have your child notice how this feels in their body. Typically forward bends are relaxing to the nervous system. Still, as with all the yoga postures, it is important to ask what they are experiencing and validate whatever is true for them with this practice.

Attunement

It's the child really feeling that you are with them that heals the most. Sometimes healing doesn't require words.

—Lisa Dion

Understanding attunement, the embodied experience of deeply connecting with your child, is crucial as you navigate the nuance of all these practices. Attunement supports us in knowing when to lean in and when to lean back, when it is the right time to share a practice and when it is time to simply hold a loving space for our child's pain. Connecting in this way ensures that our tone is authentically supportive as we acknowledge their struggle, and it can help us stay in touch with our intention to offer loving care in the midst of difficulty.

We have used the term *loving, connected presence* throughout this book—it is our attunement that supports that connection. Attunement is the magic that brings it all together. It is important to stress that what we share throughout this book is not prescriptive. It isn't just saying the right words, checking off the three parts of self-compassion, or doing the activities. This ability to be a loving, connected presence is the essence of compassion and what most supports our child in a difficult moment.

For example, we may feel that our child needs to hear us acknowledge their pain and say, "Oh, honey, that is really hard." However, with attunement we are also able to sense if it isn't the moment to say, "I am sure your friends feel that way too sometimes." Though that statement is true and supports common humanity—one of the aspects of self-compassion— maybe we can tell our child isn't quite ready to hear that yet. We can feel some resistance. If we attune by first checking in with our own inner experience, we may also notice if our desire to share about common humanity is more about making their hard feelings go away and alleviating our own discomfort with their struggles than about cultivating this aspect of self-compassion in their lives.

Children need to be seen, heard, and to feel felt. Our capacity to attune to or feel with our children depends on our willingness to embody our own lives more fully. We first connect to our own embodied experience, settle our own nervous systems as needed, and then open up to theirs. More than anything we do, our ability to be present in a loving way for our children, to feel with them, is what teaches them to be present and loving toward themselves.

Attunement is an ongoing practice. Being kind to ourselves when we feel we didn't connect with our child in this way is yet another opportunity to model self-compassion. The practice of attunement is new for many of us. I know it was for me. So please be kind and gentle with yourself as you explore this further. And remember, every moment is a chance to begin again.

9

The Power of Words and Thought

EVEN AS A CHILD, I (Wendy) didn't believe the saying "Sticks and stones may break my bones, but words will never hurt me." Words did and still do hurt! Harsh words from others, but even more so the harsh words we tell ourselves, can be extremely painful. The names we call ourselves and the things we say can be both hurtful and unhelpful. Exploring how we can use words and our thoughts—that is, our inner words—to support instead of harm us can be a lifelong practice and one our children could benefit from greatly. Noticing our inner critic and handling it effectively, including shifting that inner voice to one that is kind, caring, and supportive, can make a big difference.

If we agree that words matter, then let's look more closely at the words we say to ourselves, the words we say to our children, and the words they say to themselves in thoughts and out loud.

How We Talk to Ourselves

How we talk to ourselves and the topic of judgment and shame were already addressed in part one of this book. However, it is important to remember that how we talk to ourselves—our inner voice—also impacts our children. The analogy of the cup is once again useful: what we put in our cup is what we have to offer our children. This is yet another reminder of the importance of our own self-compassion practice as we support our children.

The Words We Say to Our Children

It is in the relational field—all the ways that we relate to our children—that we most impact them, and the words we say are one apparent and essential way we do this. Of course, body language and attunement, which were previously discussed, are also aspects of this relational field. Here we will look specifically at our general way of speaking to our children and how that impacts their ability to relate to themselves with kindness.

You have probably noticed your words in their self-talk and their comments to others. Our children often repeat what we say and even use our tone of voice for better and sometimes for worse. It can be helpful for us to practice being more deliberate in this area, gently setting the intention to speak to our children how we would like them to speak to themselves. As with our other intentions, we want to hold it lightly and kindly. With that in mind, it is incredibly important not to judge ourselves when we speak in ways that are rushed, unhelpful, or even at times unkind. Apologizing when what we said was unskillful can be a powerful use of words as it helps our children understand that no one is perfect; all beings make mistakes and can take responsibility for them.

Then we begin again. We go gently with ourselves, and we recommit to this intention because how we talk to our children—both the tone and the words—plants the seeds for their inner voice. We want to help our children develop self-talk that is kind, caring, and encouraging. Imagine the impact it could have on their lives to have an inner voice that can offer them kindness, tenderness, and compassion in difficult moments.

How quickly children take in our words became even more apparent to me at a recent gathering. There was only one family there with children: a three-year-old boy and his baby sister. The three-year-old was a bit overwhelmed at first with all the adults in the crowded room. To my surprise, when I offered, he happily sat with me in a corner to read. At one point, his little sister started to cry, and he looked over at her. I commented that the baby seemed sad. He replied in the same soft, kind tone I used while reading to him: "Everyone feels sad sometimes," a line straight out of the book we just read. In just one reading of this book, my words and the message had already started to sink in. As he shared stories about moving and having a baby sister, he periodically used phrases from the book to offer himself kindness and comfort with no prompting from the adults in the room.

Children absorb what they hear. Let's help them take in messages of kindness and compassion. Messages that say "You do not need to be perfect," "You are loved and seen and worthy," and, as this little one did, the message that everyone has a hard time sometimes. How deeply it sinks in is usually benefited by repetition, but as I experienced, even in a one-time meeting, our words have an impact.

When using any of the following suggestions and, in general, when paying attention to our own inner voice or our conversations with our children, it is helpful to notice our tone as well as the words. How we say something is as important as what we say. I am sure you can think of examples in your life where this rings true. Children are incredibly perceptive and will pick up on the slightest irritation or frustration in your voice. So, if you are feeling frustrated, irritated, or impatient, there is absolutely no judgment. Like all parents, you feel that way at times, and those may be good moments to take care of yourself before responding to their struggles.

THE WORDS WE SAY IN MOMENTS OF DIFFICULTY AND THE SELF-COMPASSION BREAK

In chapter 2 we already practiced for ourselves the Self-Compassion Break from the Mindful Self-Compassion program. We can model this practice in our conversations with our children when they are experiencing a challenging time by using phrases to support the three aspects of self-compassion individually or in combination. Our children will learn how to offer themselves self-compassion if they consistently hear us use phrases that remind them that they are not alone in experiencing difficulties and phrases that support mindfulness and kindness.

Notice what words or phrases resonate with you and your child. It is important for the phrases to be authentic and relatable, so play with the wording that fits your conversational style. That said, sometimes, talking this way can feel awkward at first. Though it is important to find words that resonate with your family, also be willing to experiment and give it a chance, even if initially it is a bit uncomfortable.

When your child is having a hard time with something, try using phrases that support mindfulness, such as:

That sounds really hard, or tricky, or difficult, or stressful, or . . .
It sounds like your feelings are hurt, or you are frustrated, or embarrassed, or . . .
I am wondering if you might be feeling sad about that; that can feel yucky.

You can also use phrases to remind them that they are not alone, such as:

Everyone makes mistakes sometimes. (We can't say this enough to our children and to ourselves!)
Sometimes things don't go how we want, or sometimes we get disappointed.
Of course you feel that way.
It makes sense that you feel that way.
I imagine lots of other children would feel the same way.

You can offer words of kindness, such as:

I am here with you.
I've got you, honey.

Can you be kind to yourself?

It's okay, sweetie (or another term of endearment you may use). I
   am right here.

Could you use a hug?

You can also offer some words of encouragement or motivation:

You've got this, honey.

Would you like to ask for help?

Who can you ask for help?

I know this is hard, and you can do hard things.

Yes, this is really hard. I wonder what you think you should do.

What do you need now?

THREE STONES OF THE SELF-COMPASSION BREAK

For this activity, you and your child can take a mindful walk together.
Invite them to find three small stones while you are taking your walk.
When you return home, you can mindfully explore the stones together,
noticing their size, shape, color, texture, temperature, smell, and sound.
Explain to your child that for this activity, each stone will represent one
part of a self-compassion practice: one stone is for mindfulness, one stone
is for common humanity or "noticing others," and one stone is for kindness. Next, invite them to assign a stone for each of the three components
of self-compassion.

Now ask your child to decorate the three stones using paint or markers, perhaps writing the words *mindfulness*, *noticing others*, and *kindness*
on the stones. Younger children can draw little symbols on the stones to
represent each component. You can give them a little mesh bag to store
the three stones, if you like.

Share that we can use the stones to help us practice self-compassion
when we are going through a hard time. Explain that we can hold the
mindfulness stone, take a deep breath, and notice the emotion that we are

feeling and also that we are finding things tough right now. We can gently say to ourselves, "This is a hard moment," or another phrase we may have used above. Next, we can hold the "noticing others" stone and remember that we are not the only ones feeling like this. We can say to ourselves, "I am not the only one," or one of the other phrases for common humanity that resonates with your child. Finally, we can hold the kindness stone and offer ourselves some care and kindness. We can, for example, ask ourselves, "How can I be kind to myself in this moment?" or use one of the other phrases we may have used from above.

The three stones can be kept in your child's special space. They can even take them to school or on a trip, especially if they anticipate that they may encounter difficulty or discomfort that day. It may also be helpful to put one set of stones somewhere very visible, like on your kitchen windowsill, to support your own and your family's daily self-compassion practice.

SELF-COMPASSION BREAK WITH THE THREE STONES REFLECTION

This reflection may be especially helpful when your child is experiencing a difficult time. They will need their three stones to support them with this practice.

THREE STONES REFLECTION SCRIPT

When we are having a hard time, it can really help us to practice being a kind friend to ourselves. We can practice a special meditation that helps us to do this. The meditation has three different steps, and we will use our three stones to help us.

The first step is mindfulness. Can you take the mindfulness stone from your bag and hold it in your hand?

Close your eyes if you like and take a few deep breaths in and out.

Now notice how you feel right now. How does your body feel? How does your head feel? How does your heart feel? Remember, however you feel right now, that's okay. You are just right as you are. Is there something that feels hard for you right now? Do you have an emotion that is tricky for you to feel?

If you are having a tough time, you can say to yourself, "This is hard," or "I am finding this tricky."

The next step is about noticing others. Take the "noticing others" stone from the bag, hold it in your hand, and say to yourself, "It is okay to feel the way that I do. All my feelings are okay. There are lots of other children who are feeling just like me. I am not the only one who feels like this."

The last step is about being kind. Take the kindness stone from your bag and close your eyes again if you like. Imagine there is a really good friend there with you now—the kindest, most caring friend in the whole world. It can be a real person that you know or an imaginary person. Try to imagine what kind of words this friend would say to you. Try to hear the words as clearly as you can.

Now see if you can become like this kind friend. Can you say some kind and caring words to yourself?

You can say things like:

It is okay to have a hard day.
How I feel now is okay.
Right now, it is like this, but I will feel different soon.
I am just right as I am.
I am enough.
I am loved.
What do I need that could help me right now?

Take some time to practice being a really kind friend to yourself, and then put your kindness stone back in its bag.

Notice how you feel now. How does your body feel? How does your head feel? How does your heart feel? Remember, however you feel, that's okay. All of your feelings are okay to have. When you are ready, you can wriggle your fingers and toes, then slowly and gently open your eyes.

Validation and the Magic of *And*

Many years ago, I was at a training and learned about the power of using the word *and* instead of the word *but*. By using the connecting word *and*, we validate our child's feelings, model identifying and naming them (mindfulness), and encourage them to understand that there is more than just that difficult feeling. You could use *and* to connect the difficult emotion to a phrase about common humanity. For example, "I know you feel worried about starting school, *and* I imagine lots of kids feel worried about the first day of school." You can also remind them that sometimes things are hard or don't go their way, *and* they can handle it—a little bit of the encouraging aspect of self-compassion. It can also be helpful in connecting to what you need them to do next: "I know you are sad to leave your friend's house, *and* it is time to clean up and get ready to go." By using *and*, we support the practice of mindfulness, an essential aspect of self-compassion, and hold it in a larger context, one that can also include common humanity and self-kindness.

As a little one, my son hated to get up in the mornings, and it was often a stressful time. When we started to use *and*, we would say, "I know you are tired; it is so hard to get up." We would then leave a pause for that validation and kindness to sink in before adding, "And it's time to get ready for school." It was amazing how helpful this one little word became in our family life. Though there was still some grumbling at times, he would—most mornings—get up without too much struggle. A key part of this practice is the pause before using the word *and*. Attunement, as was previously mentioned, is essential here. Genuinely and kindly validating your child's inner experience and giving time for that to sink in before using *and* to make a connecting statement can make all the difference.

Naming and Talking about Feelings

Anything that's human is mentionable, and anything that is mentionable can be more manageable. When we can talk about our feelings, they become less overwhelming, less upsetting, and less scary. The people we trust with that important talk can help us know that we are not alone.

—*Fred Rogers*

Acknowledging, accepting, and naming our children's feelings helps them learn to do the same. Naming emotions is a way to create some space to hold them more effectively. In doing so, we separate ourselves a little from them, and they become easier to manage. Like our own practice in chapter 2 of labeling thoughts and emotions, here we are helping our children develop that same ability.

You can support your child in generally using and expanding their emotional vocabulary by asking what they think characters are feeling on television shows or in books and then sharing the names of some similar emotions. With sincere interest and kindness, you can also gently ask your child what they are feeling at different times, not just when things are hard. If they are unable to name it, you might say, "I wonder if you are feeling . . . ," or "It sounds like you might be feeling . . ."

Naming an emotion brings the part of the brain that helps with reasoning back online and can help make a tricky emotion less intense and more manageable. Daniel Siegel, a bestselling author, award-winning educator, and executive director of the Mindsight Institute, calls this "Name It to Tame It," and it can be a powerful way to support children in dealing with their big feelings. As we continue to practice mindfulness and acknowledge and accept whatever feeling is there, we want to be sure our children know that all emotions belong. In naming and welcoming our feelings, they lose some of their hold on us. Many of the practices in this book—in particular the Feeling Friends and Heart House and Feeling Visitors activities in chapter 5 as well as many activities from chapter 8—support helping children name and welcome their feelings, as does our capacity to name and discuss feelings with our children in this welcoming and supportive way.

The Words They Say to Themselves

How can we help our children say kinder words to themselves? Imagine if the person you spent the most time with was often harsh, mean, and negative. That is, unfortunately, the experience so many of us have, especially when things don't go our way or we feel we have let someone down, made a mistake, or done something we think is embarrassing. I always tell children that we spend the most time with ourselves, and yet that's the person who is often the least kind to us. This is why it is essential to help our children cultivate internal kindness with words of comfort and care, not criticism and judgment.

THE CRANKY PARROT AND TEAM KINDNESS

Let's begin by getting to know the inner critic so we can see it a bit more clearly. You can tell your child that most of us, even grown-ups, have what is called an inner critic. To help them understand this concept, we can explain that it is like having this invisible cranky parrot. You might even use a parrot stuffed animal or puppet or make one to use as you explain this idea to children. Using props can help them to be more engaged with the concept and deepen their understanding.

Just like a parrot, our inner critic often repeats things that it has heard. Your cranky parrot may say things like, "That was a dumb thing to say," or ask, "How could you have made such a big mistake?" or say, "No one wants to play with you." It can be really mean sometimes and say things that don't feel good. Not only does it repeat what it hears but it often says things that don't make sense. Because it can be really loud, it can be hard not to take what it says into our heart. You can ask your child if they think they have a cranky parrot. And if so, what might their cranky parrot say? You can also check in with them about how their body feels when the cranky parrot—that is, their inner critic—is there. Leave lots of space for this discussion, and if they do not want to share, you can come back to this later. As it is appropriate, you can also share about your own cranky parrot and what it says.

It is helpful to get to know this cranky parrot better so we don't get carried away with its stories. We could ask them if they want to give it a name and even imagine, in more detail, what it would look like. They could make a character of the parrot out of clay, use index cards and a Popsicle stick to make it a puppet, or simply draw it on a piece of paper. Some children may want to use their imagination and decide what their inner critic might look like if it weren't a parrot. As with the parrot, they can give it a name, imagine what it looks like, and make one to have and use for discussions with and about the inner critic.

Using their inner critic/parrot craft, you can support your child to practice telling it, "I see you, and no, thank you, I do not have to believe what you say," or "I know you're telling me things that aren't true or are not helpful." There are many reasons we have our inner critic, and it is important that we don't turn it into an enemy. Our focus here is to help our children see it and relate to it kindly and firmly.

Now remind your child again that the most important person for them to be kind to is themselves. To help do that, we can start to bring other voices into the conversation with the inner critic. If you made the King-dom of Kindness from chapter 7 (see The Kindness Kingdom activity), this is another opportunity to use it. Another variation would be to make "Team Kindness." Encourage your child to identify who they might want on their team. Some ideas might be Caring Carl, Motivating Maura, Curi-ous Cathleen, Strong Susan, Mellow Matt, and Kind Katie. They can make puppets, pictures, clay characters, or even use dolls or stuffed animals for all the members of their Team Kindness, not expelling the critic but let-ting the others help take care of it.

What might Kind Katie say in a tricky moment? How would the other members of our team talk to us, and how would they talk to our inner critic? You could even put them all in a shoebox and decorate it, writing (insert your child's name)'s Team Kindness on the cover and put it in your child's special space for them to use when the cranky parrot is being espe-cially loud.

WEEDS AND FERTILIZER

The Weeds and Fertilizer activity encourages children to pay close attention to their inner voice and begin to separate out those messages that are helpful and those that may be more hurtful.

Explain that weeds make it harder for the flower to grow strong and bloom; fertilizer is like food that helps to nourish and grow the flower. You can use the phrase *flower food* instead of *fertilizer* for younger children. Give examples of something that could happen, and ask them what they might say to themselves at that moment—for example, ask, "If you didn't do well on a test, what might you say to yourself?" Next, ask if what they would say to themselves is a weed or fertilizer. Does it help them take good care of themselves or could it be making things harder? How do they feel inside when they notice saying these things? If it's a weed, do they have any ideas for possible fertilizer?

Play this game periodically and encourage them to notice in their day when they are using fertilizer for their flower or when the weeds are taking over. Remind them it is totally normal for weeds to grow for all of us, and it helps to start to notice them. We want to keep this light and playful to avoid any additional self-criticism for acknowledging they have an inner critic. For this reason, I suggest encouraging them to use a deeply kind and gentle tone of voice when naming a weed or fertilizer with this practice.

SPEAKING KINDLY TO MY HEART

The Speaking Kindly to My Heart activity encourages children to be kind to themselves when they are experiencing difficult emotions and gives them practice at some kind and caring self-talk. Cut out a large heart and glue it to a piece of poster board. If you made the feeling visitors from chapter 5 (see Heart House and Feeling Visitor activity), they can be used again here. As in that activity and the Feeling Friends activity, spend some time talking about the different emotions we all experience and give them a name. If you didn't make the feeling visitors, you can now make a cutout character to represent each emotion and glue them in the heart.

Now, using "talking bubbles" or smaller heart shapes, write in some words we could say when these feelings are in our hearts, such as "I am here for you," "I will look after you," "It's okay that you are here or feeling this way," or "All your feelings matter." Any of the words we used before when we discussed using phrases of self-compassion when talking to your child could work here as well. You could also include questions: "What do I need?" "What could help me?" "How can I take good care of myself now?" Glue these smaller hearts and talking bubbles onto the poster board around the heart.

As you do that, you can discuss the questions together. Maybe your child needs a hug, some quiet time, or to run around outside. Be interested and receptive as they respond to the questions. You can also practice using the phrases that are included on the poster board and ask them to notice how their body feels as they practice. The poster board can be put in your child's special space to remind them of some kind and caring words they can use when things feel hard.

WATERING WITH WORDS

Similar to the Speaking Kindly to My Heart activity above, Watering with Words gives children visual reminders and specific examples of speaking kindly to themselves. Using pieces of blue construction paper, make multiple raindrop shapes. Ask your child what words they could say to themselves when they are going through a hard time that would be kind and caring. Have them write those words on the raindrops (for younger children, you can write the words for them). For some ideas, you can refer to the examples in the previous activity. Have them notice how their body feels when they talk to themselves in this kind and caring way.

Draw a picture of a watering can on a paper bag with the opening at the top (you can also use another container to make a watering can) and write "watering with words of kindness" on it. Put the drops of "water" in the "can." This can be kept in the child's special space where it is a visible and accessible reminder to use words of kindness. The phrases can be taken out of the "watering can" and used when your child is experiencing a difficult time. It is also really helpful to periodically take them out and practice saying the phrases together.

PART THREE

Tending Our Garden: Integrating Self-Compassion into Family Life

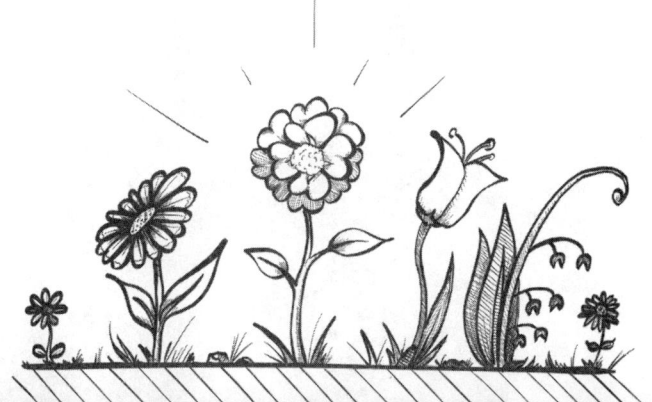

10

Nurturing Our Family
with Self-Compassion

THROUGHOUT THIS BOOK, we have shared practices and ideas to support children and parents in cultivating self-compassion. In this chapter, we will explore the important next step of integrating self-compassion as a way of being and relating to life's ups and downs as a family. The practices included in this chapter will address the final question posed at the start of the book: How can I integrate self-compassion into family life?

Growing up, I (Louise) was a very sensitive child. I felt emotions deeply, and I worried about all sorts of things. Throughout my school years, I struggled with friendships and fitting in with others and was bullied at times. As a child and teenager, I was so ashamed of my difficult emotions and experiences. I felt that I was bad or wrong for experiencing worry, sadness, and struggles in my life, and I hid my emotions and difficulties from my family and everyone else. Looking back, I feel my suffering would have been greatly eased had I known that it was okay and normal to struggle at times and to feel the way I did. I have come to realize that my experience as a child was not uncommon. So many of us have grown up feeling like our internal worlds were not seen, acknowledged, or welcomed.

The difficulties I encountered in my early years have served as inspiration for my work with children and families and have also led me to reflect deeply on what it is that children most need from the adults who care for them. Over time, it has become clear to me that what children need most from the adults in their lives are two things: presence and love. In her book *Radical Acceptance*, Tara Brach describes the traditional Buddhist analogy of the two wings of meditation practice. She writes that just like a bird needs two wings to fly, in our meditation practice we need to cultivate the two wings of mindfulness and compassion. The two wings of practice are inseparable. Both are essential and work together, mutually reinforcing each other.

In a similar way, what children are most seeking from their caregivers are the two wings of presence (mindful connection) and compassion (love and care). Presence on its own is not enough; in the same way, compassion on its own is also insufficient. However, when children receive both wings of presence and compassion from the adults in their lives, a rich, fertile ground is cultivated for their growth, happiness, and well-being. Although this book contains many activities you can share with your family, we want to remind you again that the most important gift you can give your child is these two wings of mindful presence and loving compassion.

> Most of my best parenting, teaching, and clinical work has come out of the insights, wisdom, and compassion developed in my own practice and in my relationship with the kids I work with, not in the tools or techniques I've thrown at them.
>
> —*Christopher Willard*

We would also like to remind you that integrating self-compassion as part of family life is mostly about your own embodiment of self-compassion as a parent. This doesn't have to mean practicing lengthy meditations, although it can if you so choose. It is simply about bringing a loving, compassionate presence into our moment-to-moment experience as best as we can. Every moment of your life and your parenting is an opportunity to practice.

BE KIND PRACTICE

The Be Kind Practice is a simple and effective way to support us with cultivating a loving, compassionate presence. Ask yourself at any moment, "How can I be kind right now?" If you need to, bring yourself back to "being" by connecting to the present moment through your breath, senses, and bodily sensations. Return to kindness by asking yourself, "How would I speak to and treat a dear friend in this moment?" Follow by giving yourself the same kindness and care that you would offer this friend.

Remember to be gentle with yourself as you practice cultivating these qualities in family life. Some days will be easier than others, and it is absolutely normal to find the practice difficult at times. How we show up as a parent will differ from day to day. Keep meeting yourself with acceptance and tenderness, knowing that each moment is the perfect opportunity to begin again.

Family Self-Compassion Practices

This chapter describes practices and activities that will support you to integrate self-compassion into family life. Consider including your extended family in some of the activities and practices. Invite grandparents, aunts, uncles, cousins, and family friends to join in. The key is to make self-compassion practice a normal part of everyday family life. Just as we encourage children to brush their teeth each day and look after their physical health, we can also support them to speak kindly to themselves, practice mindful breathing, and share their difficult emotions with us.

You can create a family "special space" if you like, where some of the craft activities outlined in this chapter can be kept and that represents a place in the home where your family members' internal worlds— thoughts, emotions, and struggles—are given acknowledgment and validation. The special space can also serve as a place that family members visit to practice self-compassion and as a reminder of your family's commitment to practicing kindness toward themselves and one another.

CUP OF SELF-COMPASSION

We have referred to the analogy of filling our cups previously, and the Cup of Self-Compassion activity expands on that analogy. It can serve as a reminder to continue to cultivate your own self-compassion practice and that we can only give to others what we authentically have within ourselves. If our cup is filled with the qualities of mindfulness, common humanity, and kindness, then this is what we will embody, and this is what we will share with our children simply by being ourselves.

To begin, take an empty cup and write the words *Cup of Self-Compassion* on the front using a paint marker or permanent marker. You can also write the three components of self-compassion—*mindfulness, common humanity*, and *kindness*—on the cup. Put the cup somewhere you will easily see it as you go throughout your day. I put mine on the windowsill beside my kitchen sink. When you see the cup, ask yourself, "How can I fill my cup of self-compassion at this moment?" This may be by taking a few mindful breaths, putting a hand on your heart, asking yourself what you need, saying some kind words to yourself, setting a boundary, or something else. It is also a reminder that we cannot give from an empty cup. As parents and caregivers, we need to take time to care for and nourish ourselves continually. Filling our cup is an act of love for ourselves and our family. By looking after ourselves well, we are also looking after others.

MINI MOMENTS OF KINDNESS

From my personal experience and through my work sharing these practices with others, I know that the best way to cultivate self-compassion is to let go of thinking of self-compassion as something to do and instead cultivate the practice as a way of being. A beautiful way to integrate self-compassion into everyday family life is to imagine sprinkling each day with a variety of mini self-compassion moments, or as I like to call them, mini moments of kindness. This is something that the whole family can do together. Examples of these mini moments of kindness include:

When getting up in the morning, put two hands on your heart and say to yourself, "Good morning. I love you." The whole family could also do this around the breakfast table. Or before going to bed in the evening, give yourself a hug and say, "Goodnight. I love you."[14]

Put your hands on your belly, take three mindful breaths, and ask yourself, "What would help me today?"

Put your hands on your heart, saying "I am loved" to yourself.

Feel your feet on the ground for a few moments, then give yourself a hug.

Imagine sunshine filled with kindness shining all around you. Deeply breathe in this kindness sunshine into your heart, filling up your heart with kindness. Breathe out this kindness sunshine to your family.

Put a hand on your forehead and ask yourself, "What does my mind need?" Put one hand on your heart and one hand on our belly and ask yourself, "What does my body need?" Put both hands on your heart and ask yourself, "What does my heart need?"

Rub your hands together to generate heat, put your warm hands on your closed eyes, take three deep breaths, and say to yourself, "I am enough."

Put one hand in a fist over your heart and the other hand over it. Take some deep breaths and then say to yourself, "I can do it."

In pairs, family members can sit across from one another, put their hands on each other's heart, and say "I love you" to each other, and then they put a hand on their own heart and say "I love you" to themselves.

Invite your family to come up with their own mini moments of kindness.

You can also adapt many of the previous activities in this book for your mini moments of kindness.

> Mindfulness isn't difficult, we just need to remember to do it.
>
> —*Sharon Salzberg*

KINDNESS REMINDERS

I love to scatter little mindfulness and self-compassion reminders all around my house. These messages help anchor my attention when my mind has wandered and also remind me to bring presence, kindness, and compassion to myself and my experience as I go throughout my day. Making kindness reminders is a fun activity that all the family can take part in. As well as serving as a support for our practice, it also helps create an atmosphere of mindfulness, kindness, and compassion in the home. You can make kindness reminders from stones, shells, clay, tiles, sturdy paper, mirrors, or anything else that you can write on.

Support each family member to find an object to make their self-compassion reminder. Invite your family to think of some short messages of kindness or self-compassion to write on their object.

Examples include:

Be kind.
You are loved.
You are enough.
Let love in.
You are just right.
Breathe in kindness.
Put your hand on your heart.
You matter.
How can I be kind?
What do I need?
Everything belongs.

You can use phrases that we suggested in other activities here as well. This activity can also support the intention practices presented in chapters 2 and 3.

Invite your family to write their messages of self-compassion on their object using paint, paint markers, or permanent markers. They can also decorate their object if they like. Next, encourage your family members to find a place in your home to put their kindness reminder. They can also put them in the family's special space.

TALKING STICK

The Talking Stick activity originates from Native American gatherings and meetings. Its purpose is to give members of the gathering the freedom to speak where they will be listened to with respect and without interruption from others. Before beginning this activity, it can be nice to share with your family the origins of the talking stick.

The first step is to find your family's talking stick. Perhaps take a mindful family walk together and take some time to pick out the perfect stick. The stick can then be decorated using strands of different-colored wool or ribbon. Using some letter beads, thread the words *Everything belongs* onto a piece of wool and tie it to the talking stick.

Explain that the different-colored ribbons on the stick represent the different types of emotions and experiences that we all have. The words *Everything belongs* remind us that all our emotions are okay to have and that there are no bad or wrong feelings.

Share how to use the talking stick with your family. Explain that the talking stick is a tool we can use to support us in sharing our experiences and emotions as a family. When we are holding the talking stick, it is our turn to speak. When someone else is holding the talking stick, it is our turn to listen. We don't have to say anything when it is our turn to hold the talking stick; we only share if it feels like the right thing to do for ourselves.

You and your family might like to come up with a special word that signifies when someone has finished speaking. Each person can say this word when they have finished sharing and can then pass the talking stick to the next person. If any family member does not want to share, they can just say the special word and then pass on the talking stick.

Set aside some time each week to have a family "sharing circle." It can be nice to prepare the room by dimming the lights and lighting some candles. Put some cushions on the ground and invite your family to sit in a circle. Explain the rules of the talking stick again and share that this is a time when each member of the family can share anything that is in their heart or mind. Remind your family that difficult emotions and experiences are part of life and that all emotions are welcome in the sharing circle.

SECRET SUPERPOWER MEDITATION

Taking time as a family to practice guided meditation together is an effective way to integrate self-compassion more fully into family life. The following meditation, and any meditations throughout this book, can be used in this way. Your children can also take turns guiding meditation practices for the family. You could also record yourself reading this meditation so you can participate along with other family members.

The following meditation ties in the three components of self-compassion and may be particularly helpful to practice with your family during difficult times, although it works well at any time. You can invite your family to sit or lie down as they listen to the meditation, whichever they feel most comfortable with. You also might like to put on some gentle music in the background.

SECRET SUPERPOWER MEDITATION SCRIPT

Close your eyes if you like and listen. Listen and relax.

Just like the weather, life doesn't always stay the same.

Sometimes life is very sunny, and everything seems fun.

Sometimes life is rainy, and everything seems like it's going wrong.

Sometimes life is cloudy, and everything is a bit boring.

Sometimes life is stormy, and everything seems very topsy-turvy.

Sometimes life is like a rainbow, and everything seems surprising and wonderful.

Do you know everyone has rainy, cloudy, and stormy days sometimes, just like everyone has rainbow and sunny days sometimes?

Can you tell what kind of day you're having today?

Is it a fun day, a boring day, a sad day, a topsy-turvy day, or maybe a mixture?

Whatever kind of day it is, say to yourself, "That's okay! That's okay!" If you are having a difficult day, remember everyone has tricky days sometimes; you are not the only one!

Do you know that no matter what kind of day it is, we can always practice mindfulness?

Let's have a go!

Can you put your hand on your tummy?

Feel your tummy moving as you breathe in and out.

Just notice your tummy moving as you breathe in and out.

Feel your tummy get bigger as you breathe in.

Feel your tummy get smaller as you breathe out.

If your mind jumps away to a thought, jump it back to just noticing your breathing.

That's the only thing to do now.

Feel your tummy get bigger as you breathe in.

Feel your tummy get smaller as you breathe out.

Do you know that no matter what kind of day you're having—whether it is sunny, cloudy, rainy, or stormy—you can always practice mindful breathing just like this? It's like your secret superpower! Do you know that no matter what kind of day you're having, you can always practice kindness, too? Let's have a go!

Now, if you like, you can put one hand on your heart and one hand on your tummy.

Ask yourself, "How can I be extra kind and caring to myself right now?"

Imagine there is beautiful golden sunshine all around you, and the sunshine is filled up with kindness.

Can you breathe in this beautiful sunshine filled with kindness? Breathe in kindness sunshine to your head, your heart, and your belly.

Keep breathing in this kindness sunshine until you're filled up with kindness from the top of your head to the tips of your fingers and toes.

See yourself filled up with this beautiful sparkling kindness sunshine.

Say to yourself, "I am safe. I am loved. I am just right." Then give yourself a great big hug!

That's good. Well done.

Remember that no matter what kind of day you're having, there are always lots of other people feeling just like you.

Remember that no matter what kind of day you're having, you can always practice your mindfulness and your kindness. It's like your secret superpower, and it's always there inside you.

Can you notice how you feel inside? How does your head feel? How does your body feel? How does your heart feel? Remember, however you feel right now, that's okay. It is always okay to feel like you do.

When you are ready, you can wriggle your fingers and toes, and open your eyes.

GRATITUDE TREE

Focusing on the good and what we appreciate about our family and ourselves is a wonderful way to practice kindness toward ourselves and others. As mentioned in chapter 4, the "negativity bias" refers to our brain's tendency to focus on the negative in ourselves and our external environment. This activity supports us in acknowledging the positive qualities of ourselves and our family members. Practices such as these are a way to counteract the negativity bias and promote an atmosphere of goodwill and appreciation within the home.

Ask your family whether they know what it means to be grateful. Explain that being grateful means remembering the good things about ourselves and our lives and the things that make us happy. Share some things you feel grateful for, and also share one quality you are grateful for about each member of your family. Now invite them to share some things they feel grateful for about their family members. Encourage your family to notice how they feel in their bodies as they think about and share what they feel grateful for.

To make the gratitude tree, find a small branch and put it in a jar or pot filled with stones so that it stays upright. Invite your family to decorate the tree branches with feathers, ribbons, wool, or other craft bits. Cut out some leaf shapes from paper and invite each person to draw, write, or color one thing they feel grateful for about their family on the leaves (younger children can stick on pictures). When they have finished decorating their leaves, ask each family member to hang their leaf on the tree using some wool or ribbon. As they hang their leaf on the tree, invite each person to say what they feel grateful for.

The gratitude tree can be kept somewhere in the home where it is easily visible. You can repeat this practice with your family regularly—for example, once a week or once a month, and a whole new set of leaves can be added to the tree.

You can experiment with different themes for the tree—for example, "family kindness tree," where each person draws or writes about an act of kindness they noticed a member of their family engaging in, or "family joy tree," where each person draws or writes about a joyful moment that they experienced.

WE ARE ALL FLOWERS

Begin this practice by explaining that each member of your family is like a beautiful flower. Share that no member of your family is any better than anyone else and that no family member is any less than anyone else. Explain that there is no family member the same as anyone else either. Each member of your family is completely unique and special, and each family member has equal value.

Share that just like lots of different kinds of flowers make a garden beautiful, in the same way, lots of different types of people make families, communities, and the whole world a much more beautiful and interesting place.

Invite your family to close their eyes if they like and imagine themselves as a flower. You can ask questions like:

If you were a flower, what kind of flower would you be?
What shape and color would you be?
What would your petals be like?
How tall would you be?
What would you smell like?

Next, you can invite your family members to draw themselves as a flower. In the center of their flower, they can write their name. In the petals of the flower, they can write, draw, or stick in pictures of different parts of themselves. These can be the parts that they feel good about as well as parts of themselves they find hard to like (younger children may need extra support with this). They can include things that they enjoy or are good at doing as well as things that they don't enjoy or find difficult. You can explain that all the parts of ourselves are important and deserving of our care and kindness—the parts we like to show others and take pride in, as well as the parts that we don't like so much and sometimes hide from others. Examples might include finding a subject at school difficult, being shy at parties, or struggling with sports.

When everyone has finished their flowers, you can cut them out and stick them on a larger piece of sturdy green paper. If you like, you can write on the paper, "All the different flowers make our family garden beautiful." You can stick the garden picture somewhere it is easily visible in the home or your family's special space.

You might also want to reflect with your family on the following questions:

How can we nourish and care for the flower that is ourselves?
How can we nourish and care for the flowers that are our family
    members?
How can we care for the garden of family life?

INNER VALUE REFLECTION

The following reflection is a way to explore and extend the themes of the We Are All Flowers activity and practice. This reflection will support your family members to cultivate self-worth and a deeper knowing of their inner value. It will also support the cultivation of a sense of belonging and appreciation for themselves and each other.

INNER VALUE REFLECTION SCRIPT

If you like, you can close your eyes.

Can you think about something you are really good at?

It could be anything: running, being a good friend or listener, baking, dancing, drawing, or music.

Maybe you can think of a few things you are good at, or maybe you can just think of one or two things. It's all okay.

Now can you think of something that you find hard? Remember, it really is okay to find some things hard. We all find some things tricky. That's just the way it is for everyone.

Perhaps you can think of a few things that you find hard. Maybe it's just one or two things. It's all okay.

Next, can you think of something in between? You don't find it really hard, but you don't find it really easy either.

Maybe you can think of a few things, or maybe you can just think of one or two things.

Remember, whatever you notice is okay.

It is okay to find some things easy. We all have things we find easy, things we really enjoy or are good at.

It is okay to find some things tricky. We all have things we find tricky, things that we have to try really hard at.

It's okay to find some things in between. We all have things that are neither easy nor hard for us.

Remember, you are perfect just the way you are at this moment.

There is no person in the world any better than you are—yes, nobody!

There is no person in the world any less than you are—yes, nobody!
There is no person the same as you are—yes, nobody!
We are all important. We are all special.
You are special, and every other person in the world is special, too.
You are important, and every other person is important, too.
You are beautiful, and every other person is beautiful, too.
Wouldn't the world be so boring if we were all the same?
Just like we need all the different flowers in the garden to make the garden beautiful, we need all of the different people in the world to make the world beautiful.

And you make the world so beautiful just by being you!

You can put your hand on your heart if you like and say to yourself, "I am perfect, just as I am."

Can you notice how you feel now? How does your body feel? How does your head feel? How does your heart feel? Remember, however you feel, that's okay. All of your feelings are okay to have.

When you are ready, you can wriggle your fingers and toes and slowly and gently open your eyes.

BEING LIKE A FLOWER

Being Like a Flower is a lovely way to expand on the We Are All Flowers practice. You will need a flower for this activity. You might like to take a mindful walk with your family to find a beautiful flower either growing in nature or perhaps in a flower shop. When you have found your flower, each family member can take turns mindfully exploring its color, shape, smell, and texture. Invite your family to reflect on the following questions:

Does the flower compare itself to other flowers?
Does the flower want to be different from what it is?
Is the flower ever in the past or future?

Explain that a flower never compares itself to other flowers or wishes it was different. A flower is simply itself and perfectly accepts itself. A flower is never in the past or future. It is always in the present moment. You can share with your family that we are all like flowers, too. Just like a flower is part of nature, we are also part of nature. Just like a flower belongs to the world, we also belong to the world.

Reflect to your family that a way to be kind to ourselves is to practice being like a flower. Share with them some ways that they can practice being like a flower.

Just like a flower, we can be in the here and now, and we can focus on our breathing and our senses. We can let go of thoughts of the past and future. Like a flower, we can accept ourselves as we are, and we can let go of comparing ourselves to others. We can know that we are enough just as we are. We can remember that just like a flower, we are part of nature, too. We can remind ourselves that just like a flower belongs to nature, we too belong to nature.

Finally, you can invite the whole family to be like a flower for about a minute or so. After the practice, check in with your family to see how being like a flower was for each of them.

> The heart is like a garden. It can grow compassion or fear, resentment or love. What seeds will you plant there?
>
> —*Jack Kornfield*

A Blooming Family Garden

Being human—as a parent or a child—is not easy in today's world. Things can be hard for us all at times. Self-compassion cannot take away these challenges, but it certainly has the potential to transform how we relate to both our inner and outer worlds. What a different life it would be if we all learned to become our own best friend.

The Buddhist monk and meditation teacher Ajahn Brahm teaches that the present moment is where our future is being made. In this way, we can think of the present moment like a seed. Whatever we are doing in the present moment is the seed we are growing in our lives. We hope that the ideas, practices, and activities in this book will support you in planting seeds of mindfulness, common humanity, kindness, and love.

As we come to the end of our journey together, you might pause and reflect on the following questions:

What do you most want for your child?
What would you most like to cultivate in your family life?
What is most important to you as a parent?
How do you most want to relate to yourself?
How do you most want your child to relate to themself?

Perhaps you could use the answers to these questions as guidance for the seeds you choose to sow as you continue your journey. We sincerely hope that this book's teachings encourage you to truly befriend yourself and support your family to do the same.

May your family garden bloom with love.

Notes

1. Shauna Shapiro, "The Power of Mindfulness: What You Practice Grows Stronger," TEDxWashingtonSquare, TEDx Talks, March 10, 2017, YouTube, 13:45, www.youtube.com/watch?v=IebIJdB2-Vo.
2. Shauna Shapiro, *Good Morning, I Love You: Mindfulness and Self-Compassion Practices to Rewire Your Brain for Calm, Clarity, and Joy* (Boulder, CO: Sounds True, 2022).
3. Kristin D. Neff, "Self-Compassion," in *Handbook of Individual Differences in Social Behavior*, ed. Mark R. Leary and Rick H. Hoyle (New York: Guilford Press, 2009), 561–73.
4. Kristin Neff and Christopher Germer, *The Mindful Self-Compassion Workbook: A Proven Way to Accept Yourself, Build Inner Strength, and Thrive* (New York: Guilford Press, 2018).
5. Lydie A. Lebrun-Harris, Reem M. Ghandour, Michael D. Kogan, and Michael D. Warren, "Five-Year Trends in US Children's Health and Well-Being, 2016–2020," *JAMA Pediatrics* 176, no. 7 (July 5, 2022): e220056, https://doi.org/10.1001/jamapediatrics.2022.0056.
6. Monique Theberath, David Bauer, Weizhi Chen, Manisha Salinas, Arya B. Mohabbat, Juan Yang, Tony Y. Chon, Brent A. Bauer, and Dietlind L. Wahner-Roedler, "Effects of COVID-19 Pandemic on Mental Health of Children and Adolescents: A Systematic Review of

Survey Studies," *SAGE Open Medicine* 10 (January 2022): https://doi.org/10.1177/20503121221086712.

7. Juana Summers, "America Has a Loneliness Epidemic. Here Are 6 Steps to Address It," *All Things Considered*, NPR, May 2, 2023, www.npr.org/2023/05/02/1173418268/loneliness-connection-mental-health-dementia-surgeon-general.

8. Carl Rogers, *On Becoming a Person: A Therapist's View of Psychotherapy* (London: Constable, 1961).

9. Karen Bluth, Susan A. Gaylord, Rebecca A. Campo, Michael C. Mullarkey, and Lorraine Hobbs, "Making Friends with Yourself: A Mixed Methods Pilot Study of a Mindful Self-Compassion Program for Adolescents," *Mindfulness* 7, no. 2 (2016): 479–92, https://doi.org/10.1007/s12671-015-0476-6.

10. Somayeh Daneshvar, Sajjad Basharpoor, and Masumeh Shafiei, "Self-Compassion and Cognitive Flexibility in Trauma-Exposed Individuals with and without PTSD," *Current Psychology* 41, no. 4 (April 10, 2020): 2045–52, https://doi.org/10.1007/s12144-020-00732-1.

11. Serena Chen, "Give Yourself a Break: The Power of Self-Compassion," *Harvard Business Review* (September 2018): https://hbr.org/2018/09/give-yourself-a-break-the-power-of-self-compassion.

12. Matthew A. Killingsworth and Daniel T. Gilbert, "A Wandering Mind Is an Unhappy Mind," *Science* 330, no. 6006 (2010): 932–32, https://doi.org/10.1126/science.1192439.

13. Kristin Neff and Christopher Germer, *The Mindful Self-Compassion Workbook: A Proven Way to Accept Yourself, Build Inner Strength, and Thrive* (New York: Guilford Press, 2018).

14. These activities are based on Shauna Shapiro's teachings and her book: Shauna Shapiro, *Good Morning, I Love You: Mindfulness and Self-Compassion Practices to Rewire Your Brain for Calm, Clarity, and Joy* (Boulder, CO: Sounds True, 2022).